NON-WOOD FOREST PRODUCTS

11

Medicinal plants for forest conservation and health care

Edited by

Gerard Bodeker
Chair, GIFTS of Health
Green College, University of Oxford, UK

K.K.S. Bhat
GIFTS of Health
Green College, University of Oxford, UK

Jeffrey Burley
Director, Oxford Forestry Institute
University of Oxford, UK

Paul Vantomme
Forestry Officer
FAO

GLOBAL INITIATIVE FOR TRADITIONAL SYSTEMS (GIFTS) OF HEALTH

Published by arrangement with the
Food and Agriculture Organization of the United Nations
by
Daya Publishing House®
A Division of
Astral International Pvt. Ltd.
New Delhi - 110 002

"This book was originally published by the Food and Agriculture Organization of the United Nations (FAO) as Non-Wood Forest Products No. 11".

"The designations employed and the presentation of material in this publication do not imply the expression of any opinion, whatsoever on the part of the Food and Agriculture Organization of the United Nations concerning the legal status of any country, territory, city or area or of its authorities, or concerning the delimitations of its frontiers or boundaries."

'The designations 'developed' and 'developing' economies are intended for statistical convenience and do not necessarily express a judgment about the stage reached by a particular country, territory or area in the development process.'

First Indian Edition, 2005
Reprinted, 2016
ISBN: 978-81-7035-394-2

Published by : **Daya Publishing House®**
A Division of
Astral International Pvt. Ltd.
– ISO 9001:2015 Certified Company –
4736/23, Ansari Road, Darya Ganj
New Delhi-110 002
Ph. 011-43549197, 23278134
E-mail: info@astralint.com
Website: www.astralint.com

Printed at : **Replika Press Pvt. Ltd.**

PRINTED IN INDIA

Foreword

The World Health Organization estimated that 80% of the population of developing countries rely on traditional medicines, mostly plant drugs, for their primary health care needs. Also, modern pharmacopoeia still contain at least 25% drugs derived from plants and many others which are synthetic analogues built on prototype compounds isolated from plants. Demand for medicinal plants is increasing in both developing and developed countries, and surprisingly, the bulk of the material traded is still from wild harvested sources on forest lands and only a very small number of species are cultivated. The expanding trade in medicinal plants has serious implications on the survival of several plant species, with many under serious threat to become extinct.

This volume brings together a most useful collection of papers by some experts in medicinal plants. It draws attention in a sensitive way to the huge contribution of medicinal plants to traditional and modern health care systems, but also alert the readers on the many problems and challenges facing their sustainable development, such as: assessment and management of the resource base; best harvesting and processing practices; trade issues and aspects dealing with the intellectual property rights on traditional medicine by indigenous peoples. The prospective audience includes not only foresters, rural development workers and policy makers, but also all those who are involved in one way or another with traditional medicine. The use of this document will help raise the awareness on medicinal plants as an important forest resource, and will help ensure that medicinal plants are adequately included in forest conservation and utilization programmes.

The present study was developed jointly by the Global Initiative for Traditional Systems (GIFTS) of Health (a UK based NGO) and FAO. The document is based on contributions made by many experts on medicinal plants, and has benefited from the detailed comments of several colleagues within GIFTS and FAO. Final editing of this publication was done by Gerry Bodeker and Paul Vantomme. I wish to express my thanks to all of them.

I have great pleasure to release this document, in the hope that it will serve as a useful reference for all concerned with the sustainable development of medicinal plants from forests.

Karl Hermann Schmincke
Director
Forest Products Division

Preface

Having lived amongst several of the groups of indigenous peoples of Amazonia, I have observed both the quantity of medicinal plants which they use and the efficacy of many of their cures. I have been treated by these people for intestinal upsets, parasites, cuts and bruises, headaches and other minor ailments and have personally experienced the healing powers of the rainforest plants. Since so many of our modern medicines were also derived from plants and such a small percentage have been accurately analysed chemically, it is certain that there are many more to be discovered.

Whether a wonder medicine is developed from a plant or a local herbal remedy is harvested from the forest, there are many problems that need to be resolved. Historically indigenous peoples or even the countries in which they reside have benefited little from the development of medicines from their plant resources. When a herbal medicine becomes popular it can be over-exploited and the very resource threatened with extinction as is clearly shown in this volume for some Chinese medicinal plants by He and Sheng and for African plants by Cunningham. On the other hand the development of both pharmaceutical products and the harvesting of local non-timber forest products could be of great benefit to local peoples and to developing countries when properly controlled.

This volume brings together a most useful collection of papers by some of the real experts in medicinal plants and on the issues of their exploitation. It draws attention to the problems involved in a sensitive way and reflects well the new attitudes of contemporary ethnobotany which seeks both to protect the rights of indigenous peoples and to conserve their botanical heritage. At the same time, however, this does not exclude the sustainable use of these plants. I am impressed by the wide geographical coverage that we have here and that the authors are well balanced between those from the developed and the developing world. This is a volume of interest to many people far beyond those directly working with medicinal plants. It raises issues of concern for conservationists, developers, forest managers, researchers and legislators. It is a most valuable contribution and FAO is to be congratulated on including a book of such topical concern in its series on the use of non-wood forest products. Anyone interested in the exploitation of forest medicines should read the chapters in this book before embarking on any project.

Professor Sir Ghillean Prance FRS
Director
Royal Botanic Gardens, Kew

Contents

Introduction

Gerard C. Bodeker
Global Initiative For Traditional Systems (GIFTS) of Health.
Health Services Research Unit
Institute of Health Sciences, University of Oxford, UK
fax: + +44 1865 226711 Email:gree0179@ermine.ox.ac.uk

FAO's Non-Wood Forest Products Series addresses the use of forest resources by local communities in the context of conserving biodiversity and promoting local economic self-sufficiency.

This volume on medicinal plants links together the physical environments of local communities and their use of plants in promoting and maintaining their health.

Medicinal plants form the basis of traditional or indigenous health systems used, in the estimate of the World Health Organization, by the majority of the population of most developing countries.

It is a feature of traditional health systems that they span a divers range of policy areas that extend beyond the immediate domain of health. For example, prospects for the future supply of medicinal plants impact the long term viability of traditional health systems. Training of practitioners and preservation of traditional ecological and medical knowledge lie at the core of future prospects for ancient but challenged traditions. In many traditional societies, women are the primary herb gatherers and also the herbalists. Societal changes in work and family patterns also have an impact on the nature of the traditional health sector and the services it plays in providing everyday health care to the majority of the population of most countries in the South.

In recent years, there has been a growth of interest in traditional medicine, in part driven by the interest in complementary medicine in industrial countries and in part resulting from the interests of the international pharmaceutical industry. Demand for herbal medicines in the North has led to significant changes in traditional patterns of medicinal plant harvesting and, as in the case of *Prunus africana* in Cameroon, has placed some species under threat.

Accordingly, the papers in this volume also addresses the expanded demand for medicinal plants in national and international health care and the associated pressures that this demand is placing on wild sources of plants.

A number of papers report that herbalists now report having to walk increasingly greater distances for herbs that once grew almost outside their door. As habitats for plants disappear and overharvesting for commercial uses reduces stocks of wild medicinal plant material, there is a corresponding drop in the availability of the plants used as the first and last resort for health care by many rural populations.

The pharmaceutical interest in plants as a source of medicines is less likely to raise issues of concern about sustainability of harvesting, as relatively small amounts of plant material are needed to conduct the screening for bioactivity that is the basis of many contemporary drug development strategies. However, issues of intellectual and cultural property rights have emerged as significant factors in this field.

The Kari-Oca Declaration, adopted by the Kari-Oca Conference of Indigenous Peoples at UNCED in 1992 emphasized among other points:

- o that indigenous wisdom must be recognized and encouraged
- o that the traditional knowledge of herbs and plants must be protected and passed on to future generations
- o that traditions cannot be separated from land, territory or science
- o that indigenous communities require that their right to intellectual and cultural properties be guaranteed and must include the right over genetic resources, gene banks, biotechnology and knowledge of biodiversity programmes.

Several years earlier, the Chiang Mai Declaration had noted that, since medicinal plants form the basis of medicines used by the majority of the population of most developing countries, the loss of certain medicinal plant species and reduced supply of other important plants would have a direct impact on human health and well being. The Chaing Mai Declaration drew attention to the urgent need for international cooperation and coordination to establish medicinal plant conservation programs in order to ensure that adequate supplies are available to future generations (Akerele, Heywood, and Synge, 1991). These issues are even more pressing today, after a decade of policy inertia and development oversight.

Several papers in this volume offer examples and arguments to extend and refine the debate associated with these recent trends, including Graham Dutfield's analysis of the widely publicized Costa Rican model.

Both bioprospecting - as the search for new drugs from medicinal plants and the use of traditional medical knowledge as a source of leads has come to be called - and the overharvesting of medicinal plants to serve national and international markets, raise the need for new policies which integrate health, environmental and economic perspectives.

Investments are needed for the development of appropriate conservation, cultivation and harvesting strategies which will simultaneously meet the demand for low-cost and locally-available medicines. At the same time, there must be immediate effort to ensure the conservation of diverse biological resources and the preservation and application of local cultural knowledge on the use of these resources. The important work of the Foundation for Revitalization of Local Health Traditions in India is a valuable reference point in this respect and is elucidated in Darshan Shankars' paper in this volume. The essence of a viable strategy as Shankar notes, is the full participation of local community members as stakeholders, conservers, students, educators, and beneficiaries.

Even then, as Cunningham, He and Kuipers point out in their respective articles, cultivation is difficult to establish when prices for wild-sourced material are so low that there is little incentive for investment in horticultural programmes. Market conditions here seem to be working against environmental need. De Silva identifies essential oil production and local processing of medicinal plants as an additional source of revenue generation and a potential means for making mixed horticulture programmes economically viable.

The papers in this volume address research, policy and programmatic perspectives. Most resulted from a series of international meetings organized by the Global Initiative For Traditional Systems (GIFTS) of Health (Bodeker, 1996). Other papers have been prepared specifically to round out this collection of articles addressing the diverse perspectives associated with the supply, use, conservation and trade in plants for human health care.

A clear understanding of both the supply-side issues and the factors driving the demand and size of the medicinal plant market is a vital step towards planning for both the conservation and sustainable use of the habitats of these plants as well as for ensuring continued availability of the basic ingredients used to address the health needs of the majority of the worlds' population.

Kuipers, Duke and Cunningham both address the impact of the international herb trade on local stocks of medicinal plants. As international trade in medicinal plants grows to a multi-billion dollar industry, local harvesting patterns shift from sustainable local harvesting to commercial gathering without regard to the regeneration of species for future yields. Asia's herbs feed Europe's need for herbal medicines while America's stocks of native ginseng are dwindling due to demand in Asia. There is a vast, secretive and largely unregulated trade in medicinal plants, sourced mainly from the wild, which continues to grow dramatically in the absence of serious policy attention or environmental planning.

The papers in this volume join an emerging literature - including the two recent World Bank discussion papers on medicinal plants (1996, 1997), Balick, Elisabetsky and Laird's important volume "Medicinal Resources of the Tropical Forest" (1996) and the earlier pioneer work containing the Chiang Mai Declaration on the conservation of medicinal plants "Conservation of Medicinal Plants" by Akerele et al. (1991). This volume is presented as a contribution to clarifying the many policy issues associated with the conservation, use and production of medicinal plants.

The key themes of the emerging debate surrounding the status and future of medicinal plants is the recognition that medicinal plants constitute a vast, undocumented and overexploited economic resource and that they are the principle health care resource for the majority of the world's population. It is through serious analysis, such as that offered in the papers in this volume, that future policy and practice can work to ensure that the health needs of 8-9 billion people in the world will be able to met in part by the plants that have served their societies and families throughout the history of mankind. This is work that cannot not be done.

REFERENCES

Akerele, O, Heywood, V, and Synge, H, (eds), 1991, Conservation of Medicinal Plants. Cambridge University Press.

Balick MJ, Elisabetsky E, Laird SE, (eds). Medicinal Resources of the Tropical Forest: Biodiversity and its Importance to Human Health. New York, Columbia University Press, 1996.

Bodeker G, (ed) 1996. The GIFTS of Health Reports. A special issue of the Journal of Alternative and Complementary Medicine, 2,3, 319-458.

Srivastava J, Lambert J, Vietmeyer N, 1996. Medicinal Plants: An Expanding Role in Development. World Bank Technical Paper Number 320.

Lambert J, Srivastava J, Vietmeyer N, 1997. Medicinal Plants: Rescuing a Global Heritage. World Bank Technical Paper.

Part I: General Articles covering Global Issues

Forest based medicines in traditional and cosmopolitan health care

A.P. van Seters
Rainforest Medical Foundation,
Einthovenlaan 8, 2105 TJ Heemstede,
The Netherlands.
Tel/fax: + 31-23 5280081 Email: rainmed@xs4all.nl

Abstract*

The importance of tropical rain forests as sources of medicinal plants used in traditional health systems and of raw material required for modern drug development is briefly discussed. The need for the conservation and sustainable use of these natural resources is emphasized.

Introduction

Considering the yearly loss of tropical rainforests (total area lost each year equivalent to 4-5 times the size of the Netherlands), one can easily foresee a drastic reduction in the size and quality of this biotope, with the exception of a few protected areas scattered around the globe. At this deforestation rate, the luxuriant tropical fauna and flora, including plants with known or potential medicinal value, will be decimated and indigenous medical knowledge has little chance to survive. Rainforest deforestation poses a clear threat to human safety by causing *inter alia*, landslides, floods and desertification, soil erosion and the spread of some diseases, such as malaria. The extinction of medicinal plants and medicine men, however, presents a more hidden health risk to both developing countries and (newly) industrialized societies. This article focuses on the role medicinal plants play in both modern and traditional health care systems. These plants also represent an important class of so-called non-timber forest products that provide a sustainable and economically viable alternative to the ongoing destructive exploitation of the rainforests.

Biodiversity and medicinal plants

Rainforests contain no less than 60% of all higher plant species known on earth and they provide all that is needed for human survival, including remedies against disease. Through evolution, plants have developed large numbers of chemical substances to defend themselves against insect pests and fungal and other pathogenic diseases. Some of these agents can also act within the human body against microorganisms and other causes of disease, and represent an important source of natural drugs. Their highly complex

* This article has appeared, in a slightly modified form, in *Medicine and Survival* Vol.2, No.4, 1995

molecular structures often surpass the imagination of the chemist and cannot easily be reproduced in the laboratory.

More than 35,000 plant species are being used in various human cultures around the world for medical purposes and many of them are subjected to uncontrolled local and external trade (Lewington, 1993). So far, natural products from fewer than 40 tropical species have been incorporated into modern medicine and only a fraction of the tropical flora has been thoroughly analysed for their pharmacological activity. Therefore, the annual extinction rate of an estimated 3,000 plant species is a matter of great concern as it could imply the loss of a potential drug against an incurable condition, such as dementia, cancer, influenza or AIDS. The resulting health impact on the basic needs of the population in developing countries is equally important and will be discussed separately.

Medicinal plants in traditional health care

Health care and botany have evolved as inseparable domains of human activity: the medicine man (shaman) is often regarded as the first botanical professional in human history. Whereas western medicine, as taught in most medical schools around the world, has largely switched from natural to manufactured drugs, plant products are still of paramount importance in traditional health care systems of developing countries.

In traditional therapies of certain indigenous communities, herbs are administered along with chants, dance and spiritual ceremonies to expel bad spirits and to help reharmonizing the sick person with his or her environment. Plants, however, also serve a less metaphysical role, as anticonceptives in indigenous birth control procedures or to counteract tangible pathogenics such as fungi and parasites (e.g. worms, malaria). In developing countries, medicine men and women are particularly knowledgeable about the recognition and treatment of common diseases. In Amazonia, at least 1,300 plant species are being used as medicines, poisons or narcotics (Schultes, 1979). Traditional healers are also skilled botanists and have a great talent for locating the requisite plant from the green vastness that makes up their natural pharmacy. In Latin America and Africa, this knowledge has largely remained undocumented and is handed down orally from father to son or from mother to daughter. Today's younger generations often have very different ambitions and, therefore, these traditional skills are doomed to get lost even faster than the plants themselves. This is why ethnobotanists compare the death of a shaman to the loss of a national library and invest much effort in assembling this knowledge as written accounts. Recent examples of such endeavours include *The Healing Forest* by Schultes and Raffauf (1990) which is a treatise on the health care traditions of Amazonian Indians, and *Rainforest Remedies: One Hundred Healing Herbs of Belize* by Arvigo and Balick (1994).

In recent years, traditional healing in distant forest areas has come under pressure from novel diseases such as influenza and tuberculosis (Shapiro, 1993), that have often revealed the superiority of 'white man's capsules'. This course of events has greatly affected the prestige of the local healers and has also opened the market for expensive and less necessary western drugs. Apart from the heavy drain imposed on foreign exchange reserves by these imports, the existing available and often equally effective traditional equivalents have been forced into disuse and oblivion.

Although western medicine has been integrated to some extent with ancient health care systems in Asia, it has become the dominant method in most larger hospitals around the world. In non-hospital care in most developing countries, traditional and modern systems operate independently without a clear hierarchy, whereas in rural areas only traditional healing and herbal self-care may be at hand. In these countries, there is a great demand for medicinal plants that often come from the forests. In the future, the use of these plants can be expected to increase further due to population growth and the increasing importance being attached to traditional health care by the World Health Organization (WHO). WHO's 'Health for All by the Year 2000' campaign emphasizes the urgent need for the conservation of medicinal plants (see following page for the text of the 'Chiang Mai Declaration", from Akerele, 1991). This same initiative has launched a first step toward a more rational use of herbal medicines in the Carribean, following a recent pharmacological evaluation of their effectiveness and safety (for example, the Tramil Project; see in Rabineau, 1991).

Medicinal plants in industrialized societies

In the second half of this century, 'chemical' drugs have largely replaced plant products in mainstream medicine. This development is in line with the prevailing concept of disease, the belief in human-initiated progress, and the quest for pure therapeutic substances that contain no more than one active principle.

On closer analysis, however, over 25% of all prescription drugs in the Organization for Economic Co-operation and Development (OECD) countries, and up to 60% of those in Eastern Europe, prove to consist of unmodified or slightly altered higher plant products (The Lancet, 1994). They embrace such important therapeutic categories as anticonceptives, steroids (e.g. prednisone) and muscle relaxants for anaesthesia and abdominal surgery (all made from the wild yam); quinine and artemisinin against malaria; digitalis derivatives for heart failure; and the anticancer drugs vinblastin / vincristin, etoposide and taxol. These agents cannot be (fully) synthesized in a cost-effective manner. Therefore, their production requires reliable supplies of plant material, either from cultivation or from the wild. Such is the case for the wild yam *Dioscorea composita* (Hemsl.), which cannot be cultivated and is exported from Mexico and other countries in quantities of hundreds of tons.

These few examples should make one realize how modern drug delivery depends on the continuing availability of raw materials and how vulnerable it is to the exhaustion of natural resources. This awareness is even more pertinent to clients of health products stores and herbalists, since natural non-prescription formulae may contain rare and even endangered wild plants that are regarded, often unjustly, as more powerful than their cultivated analogues (Fuller, 1991). So far, only three species of medicinal plants have been listed by CITES, the Convention on International Trade in Endangered Species of Wild Fauna and Flora (Lewington, 1993).

The Chiang Mai Declaration

Saving Lives by Saving Plants

We, the health professionals and the plant conservation specialists who have come together for the first time at the WHO/IUCN/WWF International Consultation on Conservation of Medicinal Plants, held in Chiang Mai, 21-26 March 1988, do hereby reaffirm our commitment to the collective goal of "Health for All by the Year 2000" through the primary health care approach and to the principles of conservation and sustainable development outlined in the World Conservation Strategy.

We:

Recognise that medicinal plants are essential in primary health care, both in self-medication and in national health services;

Are alarmed at the consequences of loss of plant diversity around the world;

View with grave concern the fact that many of the plants that provide traditional and modern drugs are threatened;

Draw the attention of the United Nations, its agencies and Member States, other international agencies and their members and non-governmental organisations to:

— The vital importance of medicinal plants in health care;

— The increasing and unacceptable loss of these medicinal plants due to habitat destruction and unsustainable harvesting practices;

— The fact that plant resources in one country are often of critical importance to other countries;

— The significant economic value of the medicinal plants used today and the great potential of the plant kingdom to provide new drugs;

— The continuing disruption and loss of indigenous cultures, which often hold the key to finding new medicinal plant that may benefit the global community;

— The urgent need for international cooperation and coordination to establish programmes for conservation of medicinal plants to ensure that adequate quantities are available for future generations.

We, the members of the Chiang Mai International Consultation, hereby call on all people to commit themselves to Save the Plants that Save Lives.

Chiang Mai, Thailand
26 March 1988

New drug development as an incentive to forest conservation

Natural drugs and medicinal plants, along with other non-timber forest products, already yield important economic returns (Table 1). They compare favourably in monetary terms with logging and cash cropping (Peters, Gentry and Mendelsohn, 1989; Balick and Mendelsohn, 1992), and contribute in providing better prospects for sustainable forest use (Quansah, 1994).

Table 1. Market value of timber and non-timber forest products (NTFPs)

Product	Year	Value in million US$	Reference	Comments
Vinblastin/ vincristin	1985	100	Farnsworth, 1988	World sales; profit 88%
Pilocarpin	1989	29	Elisabetski, 1991	US sales
Jamu*	1992	1000	Gollin, 1992	Indonesia, local markets
Brazil nuts	1983	216	Duke, 1988	Brazilian exports to USA
Essential oils	1983	63	Duke, 1988	Imports into USA
Rattan	1983	87	de Beer & McDermott, 1989	Exports from Indonesia
All NTFPs	1983	127	de Beer & McDermott, 1989	Exports from Indonesia
Timber	1986	6700	FAO, 1987	World exports

*traditional line of health products and herbal remedies.

The pharmaceutical industry has recently rediscovered the tropical rainforests as an unmatched source of chemicals with potential for new drug development (Pistorius and van Wijk, 1993), which promises additional revenues. Thousands of plant extracts of all continents are being screened for activity against HIV and cancer in the laboratories of the U.S. National Cancer Institute. For example, Merck Sharpe & Dome, a New Jersey based pharmaceutical company, has paid US$1 million for research rights in Costa Rica and has agreed to contribute 25% of profits made from Costa Rican plants to rainforest conservation in Costa Rica (Sittenfeld and Gamez, 1993). Shaman Pharmaceuticals Inc., a pioneer in ethno-directed natural product research since 1989, considers indigenous people as partners and only collects plant samples on the indication of a shaman. This approach appears to be more effective than random collection methods (Cox and Balick, 1994) and has already resulted in the discovery of three novel drugs. Before long, one of these drugs, SP 303, will become available as a neat monocomponent drug against herpes simplex and secretory diarrhea (Rozhon and King, 1996). SP 303, soon to be known as Provir and Virend, originates from an ordinary weed in Peru that can be harvested in a sustainable way. The expected market value may be hundreds of millions of U.S. dollars. Part of the profits will be returned to the Indian communities in the form of support for cultural and health care projects and nurseries for endangered medicinal plants (King and Tempesta, 1994). As a further consequence of this development, the prestige of the shaman will be upgraded, also in western eyes.

Conclusion

Even today, plant diversity is still indispensable for human well being and provides all or a significant number of the remedies required in health care. Forests, and particularly tropical rainforests represent vast natural pharmacies by virtue of their enormous, largely untapped source of plant material and their related indigenous knowledge of its medical use. Considering the role played by plant-derived products in human health, these resources are at the focal point of a new argument for more effective rainforest conservation. Prudent harvesting of rainforest products, however, requires ensuring a high degree of sustainability and a permanent dialogue with the native populations concerned. Medicinal plants may help build a bridge between quite different medical systems, providing the best of two worlds and allowing their practices to become more complementary.

References

Akerele, O. 1991. Medicinal plants: policies and priorities. In: Akerele, O., Heywood, V. & Synge, H. (Eds). *Conservation of Medicinal Plants*. Cambridge, UK; Cambridge University Press. pp. 3-11.

Arvigo, R. & Balick, M. 1994. *Rainforest Remedies; One Hundred Healing Herbs of Belize*. Twin Lakes, USA; Lotus Press.

Balick, M.J. 1990. Ethnobotany and the identification of therapeutic agents from the rainforest. In: *Bioactive Compounds from Plants*. (Ciba Foundation Symposium 154). pp. 22-39.

Balick, M.J. & Mendelsohn, R. 1992. Assessing the economic value of traditional medicines from tropical rainforests. *Conservation Biology* 6: 128-129.

Cox, P.A. & Balick, M.J. 1994. The ethnobotanical approach to drug discovery. *Scientific American*, June issue: 60-65.

De Beer, J.H. & McDermott, M.J. 1989. *Economic Value of Non-timber Forest Products in Southeast Asia*. Netherlands Committee for IUCN, Amsterdam.

Duke, J.A. 1988. A green world instead of a greenhouse. *Earth Island Journal* 3: 29-31.

Elisabetski, E. 1991. Folklore, tradition or know-how. *Cultural Survival Quaterly* 15: 9-13.

FAO. 1987. Forest Products Yearbook, 1987.

Farnsworth, N.R. 1988. Screening plants for new medicines. In: Wilson O. (ed). *Biodiversity*. Washington, DC; National Academy Press. pp. 83-97.

Fuller, D. 1991. *Medicine from the Wild*. Washington, DC; Traffic USA.

Gollin, L. 1992. *Personal communication*.

King, S.R. & Tempesta, M.S. 1994. From shaman to human clinical trials: the role of industry in ethnobotany, conservation and community reciprocity. In: *Ethnobotany and the Search for New Drugs*. Ciba Foundation Symposium 185. pp.197-206.

Lewington, A. 1993. *Medicinal Plant and Plant Extracts: A Review of Their Importation into Europe.* Cambridge, UK; Traffic International.

Peters, C.P., Gentry, A.H. & Mendelsohn, R.O. 1989. Valuation of an Amazonian forest. *Nature* 339: 655-656.

Pistorius, R. & van Wijk, J. 1993. Biodiversity prospecting: commercializing genetic resources for export. *Biotechnology and Development Monitor* 15: 12-15.

Quansah, N. 1994. Biocultural diversity and integrated health care in Madagascar. *Nature and Resources* 30: 18-22.

Rabineau I. (ed.) 1991. *Tramil 4. Towards a Carribean Pharmacopoeia.* Santo Domingo, Endacaribe.

Rozhon, E. & King, S.R. 1996. Shaman's SP-303 for genital herpes and secretory diarrheal disease. *Rainforest Medical Bulletin* 3: 10.

Schultes, R.E. 1979. The Amazonia as a source of new economic plants. *Economic Botany* 33: 259-266.

Schultes, R.E. & Raffauf R.F. 1990. *The Healing Forest: Medicinal and Toxic Plants of the Northwest Amazonia.* Portland, Oregon, USA; Dioscorides Press.

Shapiro, R.L. 1993. The effects of tropical deforestation on human health. *The PSR Quartely* 3: 126-135.

Sittenfeld, A. & Gamez, R. 1993. Biodiversity prospecting by INBio. In: *Biodiversity Prospecting.* Washington, DC; World Resources Institute. pp. 69-97.

The Lancet. 1994. Pharmaceuticals from plants: great potential, few funds. *The Lancet* 343: 1513-1515.

Ethnobotanical Research and Traditional Health Care in Developing Countries

Michael J. Balick and Paul Alan Cox

from

PLANTS, PEOPLE, AND CULTURE
The Science of Ethnobotany[1]

According to recent estimates by the World Health Organisation, more than 3.5 billion people in the developing world rely on plants as components of their primary health care. Just as many Europeans know of the use of *Aloe vera* [Aloaceae] to treat burns, many indigenous peoples know of some common plants that have medicinal uses. Ethnobotanical research should not be limited to discovering new pharmaceuticals for Westerners; it can also be of some benefit to peoples in developing countries.

An increasing number of nations, including China, Mexico, Nigeria, and Thailand, have decided to integrate traditional medicine into their primary health systems. In these systems, ethnobotanical research plays a crucial role in documenting the traditional health care practices of the country. Medicinal plant lore often recedes or completely vanishes in the wake of rapid Westernization. In some countries, careful ethnobotanical studies have become invaluable records of ancestral ways. In areas where the people are moving away from traditional lifestyles, particularly in rapidly growing urban populations, careful ethnobotanical documentation can provide the needed foundation for educational programs. Workers at Mahidol University in Bangkok, for example, have prepared a series of slide presentations and pamphlets to teach schoolchildren about traditional Thai uses of plants.

Ethnobotanical research can also help in the discovery of crude drugs. Only pure compounds with known structures and pharmacological activities are permissible as drugs in Western medicine, but in many developing countries the price of such pure substances puts them beyond the reach of all but the affluent. Careful clinical studies can document the safety and efficacy of crude extracts or tinctures of plants that can be dispensed at far less cost. Carefully designed clinical trials of crude botanical drugs have been conducted in Mexico and Thailand. The trials in Thailand have resulted in certification of a tincture of beach morning glory, *Ipomoea pescaprae* [Convolvulaceae], as an anti inflammatory treatment.

An area of ethnobotanical drug discovery that has yet to be developed is that of "gray pharmaceuticals"—drugs of proven safety and efficacy that are not marketable in the Western world. Decisions concerning marketability in the Western pharmaceutical industry are not driven solely by proof of safety and efficacy. To be marketable, a drug candidate must affect only one point on a biochemical pathway: compounds that affect multiple points

[1] This chapter draws on material from: "Plants, People and Culture: The Science of Ethnobotany" by Balick and Cox c 1996 by Scientific American Library. Used with permission of W.H. Freeman and Company.

of the same pathway are unlikely to be marketed because only "magic bullets" (single-activity drugs) are viable in today's legal and economic environment. Drug candidates must also show superiority over competing drugs in the same market. Thus some plant-derived drugs that are not marketable as Western pharmaceuticals may still be acceptable in the country of their origin, particularly if they can be produced cheaply. The transfer of information (sometimes costing millions of dollars) concerning the safety and efficacy of such gray pharmaceuticals from Western firms to developing countries, should be encouraged, along with the appropriate patent rights and technologies to enable the developing countries to produce plant-based medicines.

Safeguarding indigenous intellectual property rights

Historically, the intellectual property rights of indigenous peoples have not been recognised. The use of information supplied by indigenous peoples in the discovery of commercially marketable pharmaceuticals raises the question of those people's intellectual property rights and the ownership of biodiversity.

We believe that indigenous peoples are entitled to the same intellectual property rights enjoyed by other investigators. Yet in many cultures, the preservation of important habitats is equally urgent. In Samoa, four village-owned and -managed reserves totalling 50,000 acres, beginning with the Falealupo Rain Forest Reserve (where the tree that produces prostratin was first collected), have been created with donated funds, and in Belize, the world's first extractive reserve for medicinal plants has been created on 6000 acres of tropical rain forest by the local government working with the association of traditional healers with significant international support. This effort seeks to demonstrate that conservation and the use of forests as sources of locally consumed medicines are compatible objectives. Elsewhere, as in India, medicinal plant reserves are being established to ensure a continued supply of plants for traditional health care practitioners and their patients.

Cash disbursement of royalty income most closely approaches the Western concept of equity, but this approach fails with peoples who have no monetary system. For many indigenous peoples, the right to live unmolested and undisturbed on their ancestral lands is the greatest value. Establishment of nature preserves that protect both biodiversity and indigenous cultures is of tremendous importance to indigenous peoples.

Indigenous perspectives on conservation

Although small by Amazonian standards (approximately 5000 hectares), the Tafua forest on the island of Savaii, Western Samoa, is precious because of the unique diversity of its life forms. Over 25 percent of the forest plants are found nowhere else on earth.

For hundreds of years Savaii Island, like the rest of Samoa, was, in Somerset Maugham's words, "lovely, lost and half a world away." Increasing prices of rain forest timber in the early 1970s ended that isolation. An American timber firm built a large sawmill in Asau, Savaii. Lack of experience with both the forest and the culture of Samoa eventually caused the firm to jettison the project. The sawmill, however, remained in operation under various owners, and the rain forests of Savaii continued to disappear. Now more than 80 percent of Savaii's forests are gone forever: only two large tracts of lowland rain forest remain, one of them the Tafua rain forest. Because of its proximity to the wharf, the Tafua forest offered the most lucrative logging opportunity in all of Samoa. The logging companies faced only one small problem: the paramount orator and chief, Ulu Taufa'asisina.

Samoans are gentle but determined people; but even by Samoan standards, Ulu was resolute. Although Tafua is a very poor village with no running water, electricity, or graded roads and few sources of cash from the loggers, not a single tree could be cut. The villagers begged Ulu to accept the logging companies' generous offers. How else could the village pay for a decent school for their children or a clinic for their sick and elderly? The loggers might even hire some of the villagers to work for them. Ulu's stance mystified the logging companies' representatives too. They were offering the village what would probably be its only chance for economic development.

The loggers failed to realise that no inducement could ever persuade Ulu Taufa'asisina to allow logging. When his father lay dying, Ulu had promised to honour his last wish: Ulu had pledged to protect the rain forest with his life.

Ulu Taufa'asisina has paid a price for conservation that few individuals in industrialised countries can comprehend: he has knowingly condemned his family, friends, and village to poverty rather than accept money from loggers. "Five times the logging companies have been here asking for our forest," Ulu explains.

> I was deeply depressed because they put a lot of pressure on all of us, persuading the people of my village to sell the forest for a few dollars. I resisted, because I love my land and the land more than the money.
>
> The land is our lives. The land is also our mother. The land is sacred. I believe that the land has provided the culture, the food, the water, and the other things essential for my people. I deeply respect the honour that has been given to me, as chief orator, to become a caretaker of our beloved land.
>
> My forefathers had a dream. They had a dream that one day the land and the rain forest would be saved for eternity. They had a dream that the land and the sea would forever be well looked after, and not destroyed and distributed to other people. I share that dream. I believe that we can become masters of our destiny if we take care of our environment.

That destiny encompasses tooth-billed pigeons, flying foxes, and dolphins—and relentless economic hardship. But Ulu Taufa'asisina, like many other indigenous leaders, sees conservation in terms that transcend economic or political issues.

In the Western tradition, natural resources are property and therefore subject to either private or government ownership. Thus Western conservation has its roots in the pragmatic use of property; according to this viewpoint, no action should be taken that decreases the value of the resource for the long term.

Many indigenous cultures, in contrast, perceive the earth as existing not in the realm of the profane, but in the realm of the sacred, a world view that distinguishes them from many Western traditions. Indigenous legends emphasise the need to protect the earth not because it is useful to humans, but because it is sacred. The perception of conservation as a religious duty, of course, also serves ecological and cultural purposes.

Though they start from very different assumptions, both Western conservationists and many indigenous peoples recognise the need to protect vanishing natural habitats. When Maori elders became concerned about the loss of native plants used in weaving, for example, they organised a *hui,* or a traditional conference, with the New Zealand Division of Scientific and Industrial Research (DSIR). They invited both scientists and traditional leaders to discuss conservation strategies. Such collaborations, although complicated by cultural differences, have provided strong support for three positions advocated by indigenous peoples: that all forest plants have a purpose and value; that the true economic (let alone cultural and spiritual) values of rain forests and native habitats have scarcely been considered and are vastly underestimated; and that entire cultures and ways of life will disappear if rain forests are destroyed. Recent ethnobotanical studies provide evidence that substantiates these indigenous views.

Quantitative ethnobotany in South America

Forest-dwelling peoples often claim that most, and perhaps all, plants in their environment have a use. Ethnobotanist Brian Boom of The New York Botanical Garden used some pioneering plant census techniques to test that hypothesis. Working for an extended period in the Bolivian Amazon, Boom found that the Chácabo Indians knew of 360 species of vascular plants in the forest surrounding their village of Alto Ivón and that they had uses for 305 of them. They collected Brazil nuts (*Bertholletia excelsa* [Lecythidaceae]) for their own consumption and for sale, for instance, and used *Anthurium gracile* [Araceae] to cure appendicitis. Boom then surveyed a 1-hectare plot in the tropical forest and found that 82 percent of the tree species growing there had uses known to the Chácabo. When he measured the densities of plants in the plot, Boom found that the Chácabo used 95 percent of the individual trees for some purpose.

Similar studies were undertaken by William Balée among the Ka'apor and Tembé Indians in Venezuela. The percentage of tree species put to use by the Ka'apor was found to be 76.8 percent, by the Tembé 61.3 percent, and by the Panare 48.6 percent. Although these findings do not prove that every forest plant has a use, they do confirm the local people's claim that the forest plants have far more uses than Western investigators have realised. Balée and Boom have concluded that certain plant families are so important in these Neotropical areas that conserving them is essential if people are to continue to depend on the forest for their sustenance. Among these valuable plant families are the palm family [Arecaceae], the Brazil nut family [Lecythidaceae], a tropical relative of the rose family [Chrysobalanaceae], and a family that includes the hallucinogenic *capi* vine, Malpighiaceae. These studies were the first to use a quantitative approach to demonstrate the value of the forest to indigenous people and thus to promote conservation by making clear its utility.

Working in Tambopata, Peru, with mestizo people, Oliver Phillips and the late Alwyn Gentry of the Missouri Botanical Garden employed an even more detailed quantitative technique to inventory the plant families used for construction, in commerce, for food, for technology, and for medicine. Their interviews with 29 field guides yielded a total of 1885 reported uses for the 605 tagged plants in their plots. When they compared data to determine whether the age of the person interviewed affected his or her knowledge of plant use, they found that the bulk of the information in some categories, such as medicinal plant lore, was held by older people. These are the people, Phillips and Gentry concluded, who should be the main focus of ethnobotanical studies and conservation efforts. Through their use of statistical tools, they substantiated the intuitive judgements of many other workers, who perceived that the long chain of oral ethnomedical tradition was coming unravelled in the current generation. Once investigators can identify the best sources of ethnobotanical information in a community or indigenous society, both local people and ethnoscientists can make more efficient efforts to conserve such information.

Forests are more than timber: ethnobotanical valuation studies

Historically rain forests have been cut down because the simplest and quickest way to convert them into cash is to harvest the timber, burn down all that remains, and plant and annual crop for a few seasons, until much of the soil's nutrients are leached out. Since most of the nutrients in the tropical rain forest are found in plant material rather than in the soil, large-scale removal of that living material (called biomass) prevents rain forests from growing back. By using the tools of economists to analyse the value of land under various uses, ethnobotanists have found that in some areas there are viable alternatives to clear-cutting.

Researchers studying the use of non-timber resources from forests in Brazil and Peru have concluded that non-wood forest products "yield higher net revenues per hectare than timber, but they can also be harvested with considerably less damage to the ecosystem. Without question, the sustainable exploitation of non-wood forest resources represent the most immediate and profitable method for integrating the use and conservation of Amazonian forests."

In a similar study, Balick and Mendelson valued the native medicinal plant species taken by the local people from a forest in Belize. From two separate 1-hectare plots of 30- and 50-year-old forest, respectively, total biomass of 308.6 and 1433.6 kilograms (dry weight) of plant material for medicines was collected. It was suggested that harvesting the medicinal plants, from a hectare of forest would yield the collector \$564 and \$3054 in the local markets, respectively, for the two plots, after the costs of harvesting, processing, and shipping were subtracted. For the 30-year rotation, a present value of \$726 per hectare was calculated for the medicine, and for the 50-year rotation a present value of \$3327 per hectare was calculated.

This study fostered a greater understanding of the value of the tropical forest to the local inhabitants and their economy. It ultimately led to the development of several industries based on the extraction of medicinal plants from the forest for processing into tinctures, extracts, and salves. Today local Belizean brands of traditional medicines—Agapi, Rainforest Remedies, Rainforest Rescue, Triple Moon—all help to generate employment for many local people.

Additional studies to establish the net present value of the tropical forest of the Neotropics have confirmed the relatively high value (often several thousands of dollars) of the products that can be harvested on a hectare in areas where land is now priced in the hundreds of dollars or less. Critics of this method of establishing the value of forests point out that the land must be near to a market or to a distribution channel in order for the economic benefit to be realised. They state that there is probably a finite market for the commodities produced under these management schemes. Both points have their validity, but nevertheless, it is clear that in areas that have been intensively studied the harvesting of non-timber forest products has increased the income levels of local people and has stimulated the development of new industries with a local value-added component that increases returns to the region or country of origin. Such studies also tend to confirm indigenous beliefs that tropical forests, if properly managed, have far more value than as mere sources of lumber and wood pulp. Given the proven profitability of sustainable exploitation of non-timber forest products, why has so little been done to promote the marketing, processing, and development of these valuable resources? We believe that the problem lies not in the actual value of these resources, but in the failure of public policy to recognise it.

"Green" industries now promote the sale of rain forest products, such as the buttons fashioned from palm seeds that adorn garments made from Paris to Hong Kong, ice creams flavoured with exotic nuts and fruits, and rare tropical essences in perfumes, shampoos, and body creams. We can wash with soap made from tropical oils and nectars, eat cereals based on grains that once sustained the Aztecs, and drive to work on tyres manufactured from wild rubber harvested in the Amazon Basin. Like other suggested solutions to the dilemmas posed by deforestation and economic development, green marketing is hardly a panacea. The continued use of these products depends on the reliability of their supply, markets, and distribution. Key to maintaining supply is the issue of sustainable resource production.

Goods from the woods: sustainable production

Of greatest concern in the development of products based on tropical forest species (usually known as non-timber forest products, or NTFPs) is our ability to ensure sustainability. But nowadays, the concept of sustainability is used in a rather cavalier fashion. In truth, we know very little about the sustainability of any production, especially of the products from tropical ecosystems. Charles Peters of The New York Botanical Garden has undertaken many detailed studies of tropical forest trees in efforts to determine the level of sustainable production or harvest of each species. According to Peters, "a sustainable system for exploiting non-timber forest resources is one in which fruits, nuts, latexes, and other products can be harvested indefinitely from a limited area of forest with negligible impact on the structure and dynamics of the plant populations being exploited." A plant such as *Brosimum alicastrum* [Moraceae], a tree found in Central and South America that is exploited for its protein-rich fruits, needs to produce over 1.5 million seeds to ensure that *one* tree will live long enough to reproduce. If most of the fruits produced by this species were to be harvested rather than left to grow in the forest, the population would become extinct within one generation.

Too little is known about the levels of sustainable harvest of many of the internationally important NTFPs, including the Brazil nut. Some 200,000 people harvest the Brazil nut from the 20 million hectares of Amazonian forest where it grows; annually they produce around 42,000 metric tons for the commercial trade, valued at approximately $35 million, or 1.5 percent of the total international nut trade. The harvest of this nut is one of the largest sources of cash income for many of these people, and reduction in government subsidies for other NTFPs such as rubber, which grows in the same areas, has led people to harvest increased quantities of Brazil nuts. What, then, will happen 50 or 100 years from now, when most of the seeds produced by once-great populations of Brazil nut trees have been removed from the forest and sold? Quite simply, the mature, seed-producing trees that are the backbone of the population will die and not be replaced, and the resource base on which these industries are built will disappear.

What, then, are the options for the continued use of NTFPs as a tool for economic development and conservation of biodiversity in the future? Charles Peters suggests six steps for exploiting NTFPs in a sustainable fashion. First, the species to be exploited should be carefully selected, after such factors as the ease of harvesting and resilience of natural populations to disturbance are considered. A tree valued for its roots will be harder to harvest than one valued for its fruits, and the harvest of a species that produces fruits in massive quantities at one time of year will be easier to manage than the harvest of a species that produces fruits sporadically throughout the year. Once the species has been decided upon, a forest inventory should be undertaken to learn where the resource is found in greatest abundance and the number of productive plants per hectare. Investigators should then estimate the quantity of the resource produced by the species in its various habitats and by trees in all size classifications, to determine which trees in which habitat it is best to harvest.

When these three steps have been taken, the harvesting of the resource can begin, but the careful measurement should continue. The status of the population should be monitored for signs that the forest is being overharvested. People should examine the status of adult trees periodically to determine whether the flowers are being pollinated, whether large numbers of fruits are being consumed by predators, and so on. If problems arise, the harvest should be adjusted to keep its level below the rate that would threaten sustainability.

When necessary, people may replant areas that do not seem to be regenerating, clean out competitive species, or open up the forest canopies to allow more light to reach the young trees and thus speed up their regrowth. The precise measurements that Peters recommends are expensive and time-consuming, and very few species have been studied from this perspective. However, plant populations may be threatened if harvests are determined by the demands of the marketplace rather than the needs of the ecosystem. As Peters notes, "nature does not offer a free lunch." In our enthusiasm to support conservation of the natural world by focusing on its usefulness to economies, we are perhaps inadvertently dooming elements of it to extinction. Only when ecologically sound management plans based on scientific studies are developed for resource extraction will the use of those resources be able to contribute to the conservation of biological diversity.

Conservation areas and indigenous peoples

Early nature preserves were established in the tropics during colonial times primarily to serve the needs of big-game hunters or to protect watershed and timber resources. The colonial administrations created most exciting rain forest reserves by simply declaring government land to be a national park or by purchasing land from private owners, the same strategies followed to create national parks in North America and Europe.

The Mexican government owned more than 99 percent of the 528,000 hectares of rain forest, wetlands, and coral reefs that are now included in the Sian Ka'an biosphere Reserve on the Yucatan Peninsula, whereas the 100,000-hectare Guanacaste National Park in Costa Rica, an area of dry lowland tropical forest, was purchased largely from private landowners for $9 million contributed by a variety of conservation organisations, trusts, foundations, private donors, and government agencies.

The Monteverde Cloud Forest Reserve in Costa Rica, on the other hand, was created partially through a "debt-for-nature" swap—conservation organisations purchased part of the country's international debt and accepted conservation of rain forest acreage as payment. While these strategies have been effective in preserving land, they have been primarily focused on meeting national needs rather than the concerns of local peoples.

These traditional strategies create reserves that are essentially free from human disturbance. New strategies differ in that they emphasise the possibility of using the resource while protecting it from degradation. In the late 1980s, Brazil created a category of forest reserve known as the "extractive reserve," an area where local people can extract products on a small scale while still preserving a largely intact ecosystem. This form of biological reserve is closely associated with a social movement, begun in the state of Acre, which attempts to improve economic standards among Brazil's traditional peoples. The first reserves were established for the extraction of rubber and Brazil nuts. Most of the rubber produced in the Amazon Basin is gathered in a way that does not destroy the trees, so the people who gather it are strongly opposed to any destruction of the rain forest. When ranchers who wished to clear the forest assassinated Chico Mendes, the movement's most visible leader and organiser of the local rubber tappers' union, there was such an outcry that the government eventually responded by creating the first major extractive reserves, which now total some 10 percent of the entire state of Acre. Over the last few years, however, the value of both wild-harvested rubber and Brazil nuts has fallen. Ethnobotanists and taxonomists such as Douglas Daly of the New York Botanical Garden are working with local inhabitants of the reserves to identify other species that can be produced for regional and international commerce and provide income opportunities for the people who protect these areas of tropical forest. Individuals in north temperate countries are also helping to create extractive reserves. Such organisations as Conservation International and Cultural Survival have organised the marketing of forest products from reserves.

Maintaining an extractive reserve is not without its problems. The forest ecosystem may be damaged if economically important products are overharvested. An extractive reserve differs from a parcel of land that is simply public property in that a social structure is a key element of the reserve. Ideally, guidelines can be developed and rules and regulations enforced. While such rules do not exist or are strongly enforced elsewhere, it appears that most reserves are respected by the local people, particularly if they are established with an understanding of local culture and needs.

Sometimes the ecosystem of a forest reserve can be altered by protecting economically important species (or even augmenting them by strategic replanting) while other species—those whose value is not clear—are not protected with the same tenacity. Thus, some critics have argued, extractive reserves are able to protect only a portion of the biodiversity they contain. The lesson is that there is no one formula for protecting wildlands, especially in remote regions of the tropics. But in the global effort to assemble a jigsaw puzzle of conservation areas, ethnobotanical research can play an important role by helping to preserve and disseminate traditional knowledge. When this knowledge is applied, economic returns can accrue to those who make their living in the rain forest while still protecting it.

Conflicts between indigenous peoples and nature preserves

Because indigenous peoples have seldom been involved in the planning process, conflicts have often arisen between them and Western-educated preserve managers. Conflict has been particularly acute over the management of Amboseli National Park in Kenya, which is overgrazed and thus capable of supporting far smaller animal populations than in the past. "The decline of Amboseli has little to do with the large number of tourists that used to visit it or with the increase in elephant population—excuses often used by the authorities, for which there is ample evidence to refute," writes David Lovett Smith, a former warden of Amboseli.

> The demise has been brought about, in my opinion, by inept management and a total lack of communication with the local people. . . .For it was the Masai people who themselves who looked after wildlife until governments and wildlife authorities took over its management, and, from the 1970s on, proceeded to mismanage it so badly.

Implicit in the authorities' explanation of Amboseli's degradation is the view that the Masai and their herds are inimical to efforts to conserve the ecosystem, rather than potential parts of the solution. But changing such a view requires reconsideration of some of the fundamental tenets of Western land ownership and management.

Consider the differences between Western and indigenous notions of property ownership among the Turkana, a pastoral African people living in the Rift Valley of north-western Kenya, about 20 kilometres north-west of Amboseli National Park. Like many indigenous peoples, the Turkana do not believe in private ownership of natural resources. Instead, the *Acacia* [Mimosaceae] trees that their goats feed on are administered as a communal trust. Villager elders ration feeding privileges, chasing away offending goats with sticks. In Western view, such communal trusts are inherently unstable. According to most Western theorists, such resources will inevitably be degraded, and the result will be what bioethicist Garrett Hardin has termed "the tragedy of the commons".

To forestall what they saw as the "inevitable" collapse of the Turkana grazing system, a team commissioned by the United Nations divided up the Turkana grazing areas into plots, which were then deeded to private individuals. The village elders' sticks were no longer required. Soon, however, all of the *Acacia* trees were all denuded. George Monbiot argues that while the indigenous system of communal ownership of the *Acacia* trees might not have been sustainable in a Western society, it worked for the Turkana.

A new and very important branch of ethnobotany might be termed "ethno-conservation biology"—the incorporation of indigenous conservation models into wildlands management. Attempts are now being made to document indigenous conservation strategies throughout the world.

An ethno-biomedical forest reserve in Belize

Belize is a small nation with a population of around 200,000. Vast tracts of forest still cover a significant portion of the country. A recent environmental profile of Belize estimated that more than 93 percent of the country could be classified as forest land, although this estimate was optimistic, for it excluded only urban areas and large-scale farming operations. In 1988 the Belize Ethnobotany Project was initiated to inventory, understand, and conserve as much ethnobotanical data as possible in a country that is undergoing rapid change, accompanied by loss of natural habitat and the erosion of existing cultures. The project is a collaborative effort between The New York Botanical Garden's Institute of Economic Botany, and the Ix Chel Tropical Research foundation in the Cayo District with the Belize Centre for Environmental Studies, the Belize Zoo and Tropical Education Centre, the Belize College of Agriculture, and a host of other government and non-governmental organisations in Belize. This multitiered effort has linked the mutual interests and activities of local healers, farmers, students, ethnobotanists, and pharmaceutical researchers to the conservation of their main source of materials and ideas: the area's forests. These forests serve as both a classroom and a source of raw materials for local health practitioners. An ongoing inventory of species and their uses focuses in the collection, documentation, and study of traditional medicines. Collection efforts in small villages and isolated forest regions have been linked to the Developmental Therapeutics Program of the National Cancer Institute in the United States, supplying it with more than 2000 bulk samples for testing in its cancer- and AIDS-screening programme.

Supplementing the more familiar role of ethnobotany as a documentary science, the project seeks to renew interest in cultural knowledge and its transmission, particularly in the area of medical practices. It has focused on work with groups of elderly healers, most of whom have no apprentices and whose accumulated knowledge is in danger of being lost. The long-term interdisciplinary nature of the project has allowed in-depth work with traditional healers in efforts to understand disease concepts, healing traditions, and the uses of plants. This type of knowledge recovery has been described as "salvage ethnobotany".

The project helped local organisations convene four national traditional healers' meetings. The open forum provided by these meetings enabled healers from different cultural groups and geographic regions of Belize for the first time to exchange information about the medical uses of local and exotic plants. They discussed the importance of traditional healing, the central role of the healer as community health care provider, and the increasing difficulty of locating certain useful species.

In 1992 the Belize Association of Traditional Healers was formed and Rosita Arvigo of the Ix Chel Tropical Research Foundation was elected its president. Yet without plants, their work is impossible. As one of the healers, Hortense Robinson, said, "we can't do our work without the plants—it's like a mechanic without his tools. Just knowing what the name of the plant was won't help—you can't use the name to heal you." As part of the effort to conserve species that are important to the work of traditional healers, a 2400-hectare parcel of lowland tropical forest was given forestry reserve status in June 1993 at the suggestion of a government minister, Daniel Silva, who noted that Belize has a rich tradition of conservation reserves. It has reserves for jaguars, for monkeys, for butterflies, so why not for medicinal plants? The reserve was intended to provide a source of medicinal plants as well as a place to teach apprentices. Funds for surveying and demarcating the reserve were provided by the Healing Forest Conservancy and the Rex Foundation. The forest, in the Yalbak region of Belize, contains a wide diversity of fauna as well as many useful medicinal plant species. As originally conceived, this "ethno-biomedical forest reserve" would serve as a site to promote ethnobotanical and ecological research in efforts to define harvesting regimes for sustainable extraction. Toward this end, a team of scientists is carrying out ecological inventories as well as experiments designed to learn at what rates bark and roots will regenerate after harvest. Unfortunately, within a year after the reserve was established, the local government changed, and controversy arose over which group of local healers would be responsible for its operation. Various plans have been submitted to the Forestry Department and scientific experiments continue, but development of the educational and social component of the reserve's program is currently on hold. Despite the best of intention, not all conservation efforts are immediately successful.

As habitat destruction and overharvesting are depleting the supply of medicinal plants in the forests of Belize, Rosita Arvigo and Gregory Shropshire of the Ix Chel Tropical Research Foundation have started a program to develop horticultural nurseries in collaboration with Hugh O'Brien of the Belize College of Agriculture. As part of the program, the subject of medicinal plants was introduced into the college curriculum. The major goal of the joint project is to learn to propagate many of the commercially valuable plants currently harvested from the wild. The species differ wildly in their morphology and biology—some are easily reproduced weedy herbs while others are long-lived trees—so the task is complex. Local and regional businesses that depend on native plants will ultimately benefit from techniques being developed in the nurseries. The project also rescues plants threatened by development. A team from Ix Chel and the Belize College of Agriculture collects seedlings of rare or slow-growing trees from areas soon to be cleared for housing and transplants them to a "tree orphanage." Eventually they will settle the young trees in more secure areas, such as forest reserves and privately owned farmlands.

The future of ethnobotanical conservation

Many challenges face ethnobotanists in future years, particularly the rapid loss of biodiversity and the concomitant loss of indigenous knowledge systems. UCLA anthropologist Johannes Wilbert tells us that many years ago the Warao of Venezuela were highly amused when he carefully documented their traditional dances. Why, they wondered, had this man come so far to study something everyone knew how to do? When their grandchildren attempted the same dances three decades later, they turned to Wilbert to find out if they were doing them correctly.

Some contemporary critics fear that outsiders' studies of traditional knowledge is not without risk. Published reports of the use of a medicinal plant might create a demand for the resource, with riches flowing to all parties involved except the original owners of the knowledge. Others fear that if only the most sensational information is written down, the more mundane information—about food plants, for instance—may be lost. Clearly, one priority for the future is to involve indigenous colleagues in ethnobotanical research as coinvestigators and to train a new generation of people from a variety of cultures to initiate studies among their own people.

Increasingly, the local people involved in ethnobotanical research, especially the healers, are being credited as co-authors of scientific papers and receiving patent rights to discoveries that result from the information they have provided. In ethnobotanical research , anything less than equal treatment should be viewed as unacceptable.

Is there, then, a place for indigenous cultures in the twenty-first century? While we have no wish to deny modern technology to indigenous peoples, we also have no desire to see them plunged needlessly into the problems of modernity. In this, as in so many issues, we rely on indigenous wisdom. We believe that indigenous peoples, if given the proper information and granted status as equal partners, are capable of plotting their own future. And while that future will probably include satellite ground stations, kidney dialysis machines, and personal computers, we are determined that the information flow should not be one-way, from Western nations to indigenous peoples. One of the most important lessons that we have learned as ethnobotanists is that the richness of indigenous plant uses, and the dignity of indigenous knowledge systems, will not only continue to be part of the cultures in which they developed but will also increasingly grace our own.

Between a rock and a hard place: Indigenous peoples, nation states and the multinationals

Graham Dutfield
Programme for Traditional Resource Rights
Oxford Centre for the Environment, Ethics and Society
Mansfield College
University of Oxford
Oxford OX1 3TF, UK
Tel/fax: +44 1865 284 665 E-mail: wgtrr.ocees@mansfield.ox.ac.uk

Abstract

Many indigenous peoples are suspicious of 'bioprospecting'. They fear that traditional knowledge and resources will be misappropriated by an unholy alliance of corporations and governments. Trends in international law justify these concerns. Moreover, even 'enlightened' bioprospecting institutions give insufficient priority to the welfare of local communities. In response, indigenous peoples are seeking to re-establish control over their territories and prevent bioprospecting without their authorisation.

Introduction

Exploring tropical forests for new pharmaceutical leads is being promoted enthusiastically as an innovative way to save the forests. 'Bioprospectors' express optimism that they can help to implement the 1992 Convention on Biological Diversity by encouraging biodiversity conservation and stimulating capacity building in developing countries. Many indigenous peoples, though, are sceptical of existing bioprospecting agreements. As this article will explain, most agreements are based upon acceptance of two international trends which indigenous peoples feel threatened by. These are the standardisation of intellectual property rights law, and the extension of nation state sovereignty to encompass all biogenetic resources within national boundaries.

A brief history of bioprospecting

Bioprospecting is the collection and screening of biogenetic resources for industry. One of the first scientists to argue that such an activity could constitute the basis for a conservation strategy was Thomas Eisner of Cornell University, USA (1990). In 1989 Eisner and his colleagues in the International Society of Chemical Ecology adopted the Göteborg Resolution, which stated (Eisner and Meinwald, 1990):

> Natural products constitute a treasury of immense value to humankind. The current alarming rate of species extinction is rapidly depleting this treasury, with potentially disastrous consequences. The International Society of Chemical Ecology urges that conservation measures be mounted worldwide to stem the tide of species extinction, and that vastly increased biorational studies be undertaken aimed at discovering new chemicals of use to medicine, agriculture and industry. These exploratory efforts

should be pursued by a partnership of developing and developed nations, in such fashion that the financial benefits flow in fair measure to all participants.

The recent resurgence of natural product-based research by the pharmaceutical industry (Reid *et al.*, 1993:6-15) is mainly due to technological advances.[2] However, as Eisner acknowledges (1994), bioprospecting is hardly new. Since 18th century 'gene hunters' from Europe and North America have 'discovered' botanical treasures in the tropics (see Juma, 1989; Joyce, 1994), and these have generated enormous wealth. Indeed, for several generations virtually everybody living in the biodiversity-poor North has been a beneficiary of free northward transfers of biological resources (Table 1).

Table 1: The past and present contribution of biodiversity-rich countries to humanity

Pharmacy	Industry	Agriculture and food
Anti-cancer drugs: *the vinca alkaloids* Tranquilizers and heart drugs: *reserpine* Birth control: *Dioscorea (source of many steroidal drugs)* Anaesthetics and surgical aids: *cocaine, teterodoxin, d-tubocurarine, picrotoxin, madecassol, gum gutta percha* Ophthalmology and neurology: *physostigmine, pilocarpine, atropine, hyoscine* Respiratory disorders: *emetine, tolu balsam, benzoin tincture, l-dopa, sarsapogenine, catechin, camphor*	Wild relatives of plantation and other species for 'improvement'/protection Exudates: *latexes, waxes, resins, tannins, dyes, insecticides (neem, pyrethrins, rotenone)* Fibres and canes: *rattan, bamboos, jute, sisal, kapok* Edible and industrial oils: *palm oils, castor oil* Essential oils: *sandalwood, ylang ylang, sassafras, camphor, anise, nutmeg, vanilla, cinnamon, clove, patchouli, cassia* Energy plants/biomass conversion: *biomethanation, fermentation to produce ethanol, pyrolysis*	Wild relatives of crops for 'improvement'/protection Beverages, sugar, natural sweeteners: *coffee, cocoa, sugar cane, thaumatin* Beans Roots and tubers: *cassava, yam, sweet potato* Fruits Vegetables: *tomato, avocado, sweet pepper, aubergine, cucumber, breadfruit, okra* Spices: *cloves, nutmeg, black pepper, allspice, cardamom, vanilla, cinnamon* Nuts: *brazil, peanut, cashew, kola, sesame, macadamia* Animals: *chickens, wild pigs, water buffalo*

(Dutfield, 1993 [based on information in Counsel and Rice, eds., 1992]).

However, a number of influential conservationists believe that the world is undergoing an extinction 'spasm' (Myers, 1979; Myers, 1989; Wilson, 1992), and that many resources are vanishing before people become aware of their existence. This situation

[2] These advances include the development of cheap, fast and highly specific assays targeting receptors or enzymes using cloned proteins, and new high-throughput screening technologies. These permit the screening of samples more quickly and more thoroughly than ever before, and make mass screening of natural products cost-effective.

is attributed mainly to large-scale clearances of the biodiversity-rich tropical forests. Southern governments are frequently blamed for letting this happen, but respond that as long as Northern countries fail to share the benefits of commercial exploitation of biogenetic resources, conservation cannot be justified economically. Intergovernmental negotiations, such as those resulting in the agreed text of the Convention on Biological Diversity, have to some extent accommodated the demands of multinationals seeking access to the resources of biodiversity-rich areas, and of Southern governments wishing to control what they regard as *their* biogenetic assets. Unfortunately, indigenous peoples have tended to be marginalised from these debates, as they are from by the types of partnership promoted by many bioprospecting enthusiasts.

The Convention on Biological Diversity and the General Agreement on Tariffs and Trade

The Convention on Biological Diversity (CBD) came into force in 1993 and has been ratified by over 160 countries. There are three main objectives (Article 1):

- the conservation of biological diversity
- the sustainable use of its components
- the fair and equitable sharing of the benefits arising out of the utilization of genetic resources

Agreeing a text acceptable to governments in the biodiversity-poor North and the multinational companies on one side, and the Southern governments on the other, proved to be a difficult and contentious process. The latter countries together possess most of the planet's biological wealth but require greater scientific, technological and financial capacities to exploit it. The multinationals wanted continued free access to biological resources; Southern governments demanded technology transfers and benefit-sharing as conditions for access. To some extent Southern governments prevailed. Nevertheless, only the United States refused to sign at the Earth Summit, the other Northern countries deciding that it was an agreement they could live with, as did most multinationals (*Note from the editor*: The USA have in the mean time signed the CBD Agreement, but it has not (yet) been ratified by their Congress). In many ways, then, the CBD is a framework agreement setting out the terms on which the world's biogenetic wealth is to be shared out between nation states in the South and industrial concerns mostly in the North, but with some potentially far-reaching concessions to indigenous peoples and local communities.[3] [4]Thus, while the sovereignty of nation states is now extended by treaty to all genetic resources within their borders, the intellectual property rights of corporations were recognised in the final version of the CBD, albeit in somewhat ambiguous language. Brief reviews of these developments explain why indigenous peoples feel threatened by them.

---

[3] Referred to in the CBD as 'indigenous and local communities embodying traditional lifestyles'. Omission of the word 'peoples' was deliberate. This is because use of the term 'indigenous peoples' implies the right to self-determination. Many governments fear that acceptance of indigenous peoples' right to self-determination would threaten the integrity of the nation states they govern.

[4] Articles 8(j) and 10(c) are particularly favourable to indigenous peoples, but only if governments implement their provisions in good faith.

National sovereignty
According to Article 15:

> Recognizing the sovereign rights of States over their natural resources, their authority to determine access to genetic resources rests with the national governments and is subject to national legislation.

Until recently, genetic resources have been considered as part of the common heritage of humankind. Given the widely disparate abilities of countries to exploit these resources profitably, it was understandable that developing countries would wish to challenge this assumption. However, this extension of the domain of the nation state is highly problematic for indigenous peoples,[5] because it appears to contradict international human rights law, according to which 'all peoples may, for their own ends, freely dispose of their natural wealth and resources'.[6] Indigenous peoples fear that governments which enact legislation to implement the CBD will apply this principle unrestrictedly, and thereby violate their territorial integrity and resource rights (IAI-TPTF, 1996).

Intellectual Property Rights
Developing countries in recent years have been put under tremendous pressure to adopt intellectual property rights (IPR) regimes that accord with the standards which now prevail in North America, Europe and Japan. Discussions on the standardisation of IPR have taken place mainly during the Uruguay Round of the General Agreement on Tariffs and Trade (GATT), although the CBD is another important forum where IPR has been debated.

The Uruguay Round culminated in an international agreement commonly known as the 1994 GATT Final Act, which was signed in 1994 by 124 governments. It includes the Agreement on Trade-Related Aspects of Intellectual Property Rights (TRIPs). During negotiations the United States and several other Northern countries demanded protection for biotechnology products and processes in the broadest possible sense, including the patenting of life-forms. As a result, although members may exclude from patentability 'plants and animals other than microorganisms, and essentially biological processes for the production of plants or animals other than non-biological and microbiological processes' (Article 27.3 (b)), TRIPs does not easily allow countries to prohibit the patenting of all life-forms, whether on moral or other grounds. Therefore, patenting of genetically-modified organisms and even human genetic material will probably be permitted by more and more countries. Indigenous peoples are outspoken in their opposition to such patents, considering them to be violations of the sanctity of life and contrary to their moral beliefs.

Despite certain ambiguities, the CBD tends also to support corporate IPR. Thus, Article 16 on Access to and Transfer of Technology, states in part:

---

[5] Earlier international agreements have proclaimed the principle that nation states have sovereign rights over all natural resources, but the CBD is the first treaty that specifically refers to *genetic resources* (Glowka *et al*, 1994: 76).
[6] Article 1.2 of both the International Covenant on Economic, Social and Cultural Rights and the International Covenant on Civil and Political Rights.

> In the case of technology subject to patents and other intellectual property rights, such access and transfer [of technology including biotechnology] shall be provided on terms which recognize and are consistent with the adequate and effective protection of intellectual property rights.

While compliance with GATT-TRIPs and the CBD requires states to implement domestic legislation consistent with their provisions, a potential conflict exists. Implementing GATT 1994 will tend to harmonize IPR law, while national legislation to implement the CBD in biodiversity-rich countries is likely to link access to biogenetic resources to expanded nation state rights, and perhaps indigenous rights, too. Two important and inter-linked issues arise here: the possibility of adapting IPR regimes so they can protect indigenous knowledge, and the question of intellectual and biological 'piracy'.

Conventionally, IPR are conferred upon individuals and corporate entities, but not upon communities. While intellectual property law can protect inventions of companies based upon the knowledge of local communities, the community knowledge itself cannot be protected. Furthermore, in the case of patents the geographic location of the source of the raw material used for the 'invention' has no bearing on the decision to accept or reject a patent application. These features of patents effectively support the act of 'biopiracy' in which indigenous peoples and local communities have their knowledge and resources taken and used without their authorisation by corporations and governments without their prior agreement. One controversial instance of this is the case of the neem tree (*Azadirachta indica*), which has been used for centuries by Indian farming communities for numerous purposes, including protecting crops from insect pests. Two companies in the United States have patents for derivatives of the active principle without having compensated local farmers for their knowledge and prior use of the tree. It is estimated that the global market for neem-based bio-insecticides will reach US$ 50 million per annum by the year 2000 (AgBiotechnology News, 1993 [in RAFI, 1994:49]).

Indigenous perspectives

Given the sources of knowledge in such cases as neem, the fairness of IPR law is being questioned by indigenous peoples. The Draft UN Declaration on the Rights of Indigenous Peoples expresses the concerns, demands and aspirations of hundreds of indigenous peoples' organisation around the world. Article 29 states that:

> Indigenous peoples are entitled to the recognition of the full ownership, control and protection of their cultural and intellectual property. They have the right to special measures to control, develop and protect their sciences, technologies and cultural manifestation, including human and other genetic resources, seeds, medicines, knowledge of the properties of fauna and flora, oral traditions, literatures, designs and visual and performing arts.

Evidently, indigenous peoples interpret their cultural and intellectual property broadly, so that these encompass much more than knowledge, but also their cultural heritage, their biological resources, and even their cells and DNA.

In fact, indigenous peoples have their own regimes to regulate access to and control over knowledge and resources that are often more sophisticated than those based on IPR or national sovereignty. According to the North American indigenous peoples' organisation, the Four Directions Council (1996):

> Indigenous peoples possess their own locally-specific systems of jurisprudence with respect to the classification of different types of knowledge, proper procedures for acquiring and sharing knowledge, and the rights and responsibilities which attach to possessing knowledge, all of which are embedded uniquely in each culture and its language.

For this reason, the Four Directions Council argues that:

> Any attempt to devise uniform guidelines for the recognition and protection of indigenous peoples' knowledge runs the risk of collapsing this rich jurisprudential diversity into a single 'model' that will not fit the values, conceptions or laws of *any* indigenous society. A better approach ... would be for the international community to agree that traditional knowledge must be acquired and used in conformity with the customary laws of the peoples concerned.

This perspective has limited support in the CBD, which, in Article 10(c) requires contracting parties to:

> Protect and encourage customary use of biological resources in accordance with traditional cultural practices that are compatible with conservation or sustainable use requirements.

For indigenous peoples, then, protection of knowledge and resources, and continuation of customary law and practice, are central to maintenance of their cultural identity. Therefore, control over these is an aspect of human rights. This needs to be understood by all governments, companies and other institutions before they enter into negotiations for the use of biogenetic resources on the territories of indigenous peoples. These negotiations should certainly involve indigenous peoples. Often they do not. The following case, despite a generally favourable image, has attracted criticism for failing to accommodate local needs and concerns.

The National Biodiversity Institute (INBIO)

The National Biodiversity Institute of Costa Rica is frequently hailed as a model bioprospecting institution, and its agreements with pharmaceutical companies are regarded as examples for other countries to follow.[7] It is true that INBio's activities and

[7] Not only have several developing countries expressed admiration for INBio: Yellowstone National Park in the United States is considering following the example of INBio as a means to generate income. This idea was apparently inspired by a missed opportunity to share the benefits of a patented invention known as polymerase chain reaction technology, which is based on an enzyme in a bacterium found in the park. The patent is owned by Hoffmann- La Roche, and has been highly profitable for the company, generating sales of over US$100 million per annum (Iwu, 1996:79; Mukerjee, 1996).

collaborations have some positive features, including capacity building and benefit-sharing. In other respects, INBio and its agreements are inappropriate for other countries and may be inappropriate for Costa Rica, too.

INBio is a private non-profit organisation which was established in 1989 with the blessing of the government. Its main objectives are to carry out a species inventory of the country -- which is estimated to have 4% of the world's biological diversity -- and to explore the commercial potential of the country's biological resources.

Costa Rica's 1992 *Conservation of Wildlife Law* [8] (Laird, 1995; Salazar and Cabrera, 1996) declares national sovereignty over the biological diversity of the country. This is not equivalent to nationalisation of all biogenetic resources in the country.[9] Nevertheless, the State has the exclusive right to grant permits to investigate, collect and exploit the country's biological diversity in the publicly-owned conservation areas, which make up 25% of the whole country. The Ministry of Natural Resources, Energy and Mines (MIRENEM) is authorised to grant bioprospecting permits in these areas, and INBio has such a permit.

INBio's first and best known agreement with a multinational company was the one with Merck, which began in 1991 and has been renewed up to the present. Merck gave INBio an advance payment of US$1 million, equipment for an extraction laboratory, and a guarantee of royalties in case a product is derived from any of the extracts (of plant and insect specimens) which INBio will transfer to Merck. 50% of the royalties will go to the government's National Parks Fund through MIRENEM.

The agreement has certain positive aspects. First, the advance payment, which is not a common feature of such agreements; second, INBio's freedom to supply extracts to other companies, including those given to Merck if two years have elapsed since Merck received them; third, INBio has control over taxonomic information on all its samples. Thus, if an extract shows promise for Merck to continue its research it will have to approach INBio again to obtain more material.

However, before promoting the Costa Rican approach as a model, certain points merit consideration:

1) The government has granted INBio prospecting rights to explore lands and biogenetic resources over which the State has jurisdiction. Although Costa Rica is more culturally homogeneous than its neighbours indigenous peoples exist whose inalienable rights to lands and resources pre-date the existence of the country. Therefore if indigenous peoples are not parties to negotiations, an argument can be made that both the government and INBio are effectively usurping the territorial and resource rights of indigenous peoples.

2) The government and INBio are the beneficiaries of the Merck agreement. The only way that local communities appear to gain in any direct sense is through the training of a small number of local 'parataxonomists'. Furthermore, INBio will not contribute at all to

---

[8] Staff of INBio assisted in the drafting of this law.

[9] Under the Law, all wild animals are 'national patrimony', while plants and genetic resources are viewed as 'public interest' (Laird, 1995:12).

revitalising local knowledge traditions because it professes to have no interest at all in such knowledge. Nor, one can only conclude, in the cultural diversity that underpins such traditions. According to Maurice Iwu, a prominent Nigerian scientist (in Dutfield, 1994):

> The kind of deal that was done in Costa Rica cannot be done in Nigeria... The kind of deal that India and Nigeria [etc.] will negotiate has to recognise the multi-ethnic nature of our own societies.

3) A company like Merck will tend to seek cures for therapeutic groups that are major concerns in developed countries, but which may be relatively less important in developing countries where other diseases and infections take higher priority. According to Iwu (in Baker *et al.*, 1995:1343):

> Screening strategies should include parasitic infections and diseases (e.g., malaria) to aid in the search for new treatments for diseases of primary concern to source country inhabitants, and proper objectives should not be limited to the generation of pure chemical isolates as pharmaceutical leads, but should include the standardization of phytomedicines for the benefit of traditional healers and their patients. The inclusion of such measures will contribute to an improvement of the quality of life of source country inhabitants.

Indigenous initiatives for self-determination of bioprospecting rules

Indigenous peoples are concerned that bioprospecting expeditions, even those carried out with good intentions, will infringe their rights. To a large extent, the rules of the game are those of multinationals and nation states, and indigenous peoples still find it difficult to get their voices heard. In response, a growing number of groups, such as the Kuna of Panama, the Awa of Ecuador and the Inuit of the Arctic have developed their own regulations which visiting scientists must adhere to (Laird, 1995; Posey, Dutfield and Plenderleith, 1995; Posey and Dutfield, 1996). In India local communities are setting up community registers of local knowledge of biodiversity to revitalise traditional knowledge systems for the benefit of future generations and to protect them from piracy (FRLHT, 1995; Bhatia and Khotari, 1996; Dutfield and Ghate, 1997). Such initiatives are being carried out independently of governments and companies. Other indigenous peoples have declared their opposition to bioprospecting. Participants at the UN Development Programme-sponsored Regional Consultation on Indigenous Peoples' Knowledge and Intellectual Property Rights held in April 1995, called for a moratorium on bioprospecting in the Pacific region and urged indigenous peoples:

> not to co-operate in bioprospecting activities until appropriate protection mechanisms are in place.

Indigenous peoples demand that their right to self-determination be recognised *before* they are prepared to enter into negotiations over access to their territories and resources. Given the vital role indigenous peoples play in the conservation of biodiversity it is vital for us all that national laws to implement the CBD *and* GATT be enacted which uphold this right.

References

Baker, J.T., Borris, R.P., Carté, B., Cordell, G.A., Cragg, G.M., Gupta, M.P., Iwu, M.M., Madulid, D.R. & Tyler, V.E. 1995. Natural product drug discovery and development: new perspectives on international collaboration. *Journal of Natural Products* 58:(9) 1325-1357.

Bhatia, S. & A. Kothari, A. 1996. Community register for documenting local uses of biological diversity. *Bulletin of the Working Group on Traditional Resource Rights* 2: 9-10.

Counsel, S. & Rice, T. eds. 1992. *The Rainforest Harvest: Sustainable Strategies for Saving the Tropical Forests: Proceedings of and International Conference Held at the Royal Geographical Society*. London: Friends of the Earth.

Dutfield, G. 1993. *Conservation of the Tropical Forests and the Pharmaceutical Industry*. Unpublished MPhil dissertation. Cambridge, Department of Geography, University of Cambridge.

Dutfield, G. 1994. *Report on the Fourth Congress of Ethnobiology*. Oxford, UK; Working Group on Traditional Resource Rights.

Dutfield, G. & Ghate, U. 1997. Implementing Article 8(j) of the CBD through peoples' biodiversity registers. *Bulletin of the Working Group on Traditional Resource Rights* 4: 14-16.

Eisner, T. 1990. Prospecting for nature's riches. *Issues in Science and Technology* 6: (2) 31-34.

Eisner, T. 1994. Chemical prospecting: a global imperative. *Proceedings of the American Philosophical Society* 138: 385.

Eisner, T. & Meinwald, J. 1990. The Göteborg Resolution. *Chemoecology* 1:(1) 38.

Foundation for the Revitalisation of Local Health Traditions 1995. *Beyond the Biodiversity Convention: Empowering the Eco-system People*. Bangalore, India; FRLHT.

Four Directions Council 1996. *Forests, Indigenous Peoples and Biodiversity: Contribution of the Four Directions Council*. Submission to the Secretariat for the Convention on Biological Diversity. Lethbridge, Canada, Four Directions Council.

Glowka, L., Burhenne-Guilmin, F. & Synge, H., in collaboration with McNeely, J.A. & Gündling 1994. *A Guide to the Convention on Biological Diversity*. IUCN Environmental Policy & Law Paper No. 30. Gland, Switzerland & Cambridge, UK; IUCN-The World Conservation Union.

International Alliance of Indigenous-Tribal Peoples of the Tropical Forests 1996. *The Biodiversity Convention: The concerns of Indigenous Peoples*. London, UK; IAI-TPTF.

Iwu, M.M. 1996. Implementing the Biodiversity Treaty: how to make international co-operative agreements work. *Trends in Biotechnology*,Joyce, C. 1994. *Earthly Goods: Medicine-Hunting in the Rainforest*. Boston, USA; Little, Brown and Co.

Juma, C. 1989. *The Gene Hunters: Biotechnology and the Scramble for Seeds*. Princeton, NJ, USA; Princeton University Press.

Laird, S.A. 1995. *Access controls for genetic resources*. Gland, Switzerland; World Wide Fund for Nature.

Mukerjee, M. 1996. Sowing where you reap. *Scientific American* 274: (5) 15-17.

Myers, N. 1979. *The Sinking Ark: A New Look at the Problem of Disappearing Species*. Oxford, UK; Pergamon Press.

Myers, N. 1989. A major extinction spasm: predictable and inevitable? In Western, D. & Pearl, M.C., eds., *Conservation for the Twenty-first Century*. Oxford, UK; Oxford University Press.

Posey, D.A. & Dutfield, G. 1996. *Beyond Intellectual Property: Toward Traditional Resource Rights for Indigenous Peoples and Local Communities*. Ottawa, Canada; International Development Research Centre.

Posey, D.A., Dutfield, G. & Plenderleith, K. 1995. Collaborative research and intellectual property rights. *Biodiversity and Conservation* 4: (8) 892-902.

Reid, W.V., Laird, S.A. Meyer, C.A., Gámez, R. Sittenfeld, A. Janzen, D.H., Gollin M.A. & Juma, C., eds. 1993. *Biodiversity Prospecting: Using Genetic Resources for Sustainable Development*. Washington, DC, USA; World Resources Institute.

Rural Advancement Foundation International 1994. *Conserving Indigenous Knowledge: Integrating Two Systems of Innovation* (Commissioned by the United Nations Development Programme). New York, USA; UNDP.

Salazar, R. & Cabrera, J.A. 1996. Derechos de propiedad intelectual en Costa Rica a la luz del Convención sobre Diversidad Biológica. *Journal of Ethnopharmacology* 51; 177-193.

Wilson, E.O. 1992. *The Diversity of Life*. Cambridge, Mass., USA; Belknap Press.

Industrial utilization of medicinal plants in developing countries

Tuley De Silva
Chemical Industries Branch
Industrial Sectors and Environment Division
United Nations Industrial Development Organization
P O Box 300
A-1400 Vienna, Austria
Fax: ++43 1 232156 Email: TDE-SILVA@unido.org

Abstract

The majority of the rural people in developing countries use plant based traditional medicines for health care. These are still produced using age old methods which can affect their quality, stability and efficacy. Resurgence of interest in green products in the industrialised countries has created an expanding market for plant based products that could be produced by developing countries to be competitive provided the quality and safety specifications could be satisfied. The constraints for the development of such industries in developing countries and the requirements for overcoming these have been identified. The possibilities for value addition, processing and product improvement, and technical assistance needs of developing countries for the industrial utilization of medicinal plants are indicated.

Introduction

Most developing countries are endowed with vast resources of medicinal and aromatic plants. These plants have been used over the millennia for human welfare in the promotion of health and as drugs and fragrance materials. This close relationship between man and his environment continues even today as a large proportion of people in developing countries still live in rural areas. Furthermore, these people are precluded from the luxury of access to modern therapy, mainly for economic reasons.

About 80% of the population of many developing countries still use traditional medicines for their health care. Modern pharmacopoeia still contain at least 25% drugs derived from plants and many others which are synthetic analogues built on prototype compounds isolated from plants. China, India, Sri Lanka and a few other countries have officially recognized the use of traditional medicines in their health care delivery systems.

A major factor impeding the development of the medicinal plant based industries in developing countries has been the lack of information on the social and economic benefits that could be derived from the industrial utilization of medicinal plants. Except for the use of these plants for local health care needs, not much information has been available on their market potential and trading possibilities. As a result, the real potential of these plants has not been exploited by the governments or entrepreneurs.

The demands of the majority of the people in developing countries for medicinal plants have been met by indiscriminate harvesting of spontaneous flora including those in forests. As a result many plant species have become extinct and some are endangered. It is therefore necessary that systematic cultivation of medicinal plants be introduced in order to conserve biodiversity and protect threatened species. Systematic cultivation of these plants could only be initiated if there is a continuous demand for the raw materials. It is therefore necessary to establish processing facilities preferably in the vicinity of cultivations in order to create a demand and assure farmers of the sale of raw material. Thus cultivation and processing should be started simultaneously. In cases where parts of mature plants from forests are to be harvested, sustainable harvesting techniques are needed to protect these plants.

The promotion and development of processing of plant-based products have been given a fresh impetus due to certain ground realities:

- Green consumerism and the current resurgence of interest in the use of "Naturals" in developed countries.
- Free market economy bringing in more openness and expanding markets and demand for new resources, materials and products.
- A growing acceptability of the social responsibility of minimizing socio-economic inequalities in favour of rural people resulting in creating additional job and income opportunities for poor people.
- Poor economic conditions in developing countries restricting import, thereby placing increased reliance on medicines using local plant resources.
- Increasing awareness regarding biodiversity conservation and the sustainable and protective use of plant resources.
- Search for new phytopharmaceuticals for the prevention and cure of deadly diseases such as cancer and AIDS.

In 1981, the United Nations Industrial Development Organization (UNIDO) established a programme for the systematic utilization of this renewable natural resource for the benefit of the populace of developing countries. The programme aims for initiating development projects for increasing the industrial output of developing countries in the field of locally-used herbal drugs and phytopharmaceuticals which affect the economies of both developing and developed countries.

Some of the constraints associated with the processing of medicinal plants which may result in reducing their competitiveness in global markets and which have to be remedied are:

- Poor agricultural practices
- Poor harvesting (indiscriminate) and post-harvest treatment practices
- Lack of research on development of high-yielding varieties, domestication etc.
- Poor propagation methods
- Inefficient processing techniques leading to low yields and poor quality products
- Poor quality control procedures
- High energy losses during processing
- Lack of current good manufacturing practices

- Lack of R & D on product and process development
- Difficulties in marketing
- Lack of local market for primary processed products
- Lack of trained personnel and equipment
- Lack of facilities to fabricate equipment locally
- Lack of access to latest technological and market information

Systematic cultivation of many medicinal plants needs specific cultural practices and agronomical requirements. These are species-specific and are not only dependent on soil, water and climatic conditions. Hence research and development work has to be done to formulate Good Agricultural Practices which will include proper selection and identification, propagation methods, cultivation techniques, harvesting, step-wise quality control of raw material up to processing stage, post-harvest treatment, storage and safety. These aspects have to be incorporated into protocols for the cultivation of medicinal plants.

Organic farming is another practice that is gaining wide acceptance as world demand particularly in developed countries for organically grown crops is rapidly on the increase. Farmers have to be trained in all aspects of organic farming of medicinal plants and herbs including obtaining certification from associations that do the monitoring starting from cultivation to final harvesting. Organic farming which is labour-intensive gives the developing countries the comparative advantage to be competitive.

Process technology

Traditional medicines - Modern technology

The medicines for internal use prepared in the traditional manner involve simple methods such as hot- or cold-water extraction, expression of juice after crushing, powdering of dried material, formulation of powder into pastes via such a vehicle as water, oil or honey, and even fermentation after adding a sugar source. The range of products that could be obtained from medicinal plants is given in Figure 1.

Traditional herbal medicines were produced using age old methods by the practitioner him/herself who was able to identify the correct plant species. This practice of the traditional practitioner dispensing his own medicines is being gradually shifted to herbal drug stores which are profit-oriented. As a result, there is no guarantee of the authenticity and quantity of plant material used in the preparations. The quality of traditional medicines so produced vary widely and may not even be effective. Therefore, there is a need to select proper and appropriate technologies for the industrial production of traditional medicines such that the effectiveness of the preparation is maintained. Traditional methods used have many disadvantages which could be corrected by selecting the suitable technologies. It has to be stated that the traditional methods were dependent on the status of technology that was available at that time. It therefore follows that these can be modified and improved using the technologies available today to make them more effective, stable, reproducible, controlled and in dosage forms that can easily be transported or taken to office.

Hence the introduction of appropriate, simple and low-cost technologies should be encouraged maintaining as much as possible the labour-intensive nature of such activities,

Industrial Uses of Medicinal Plants

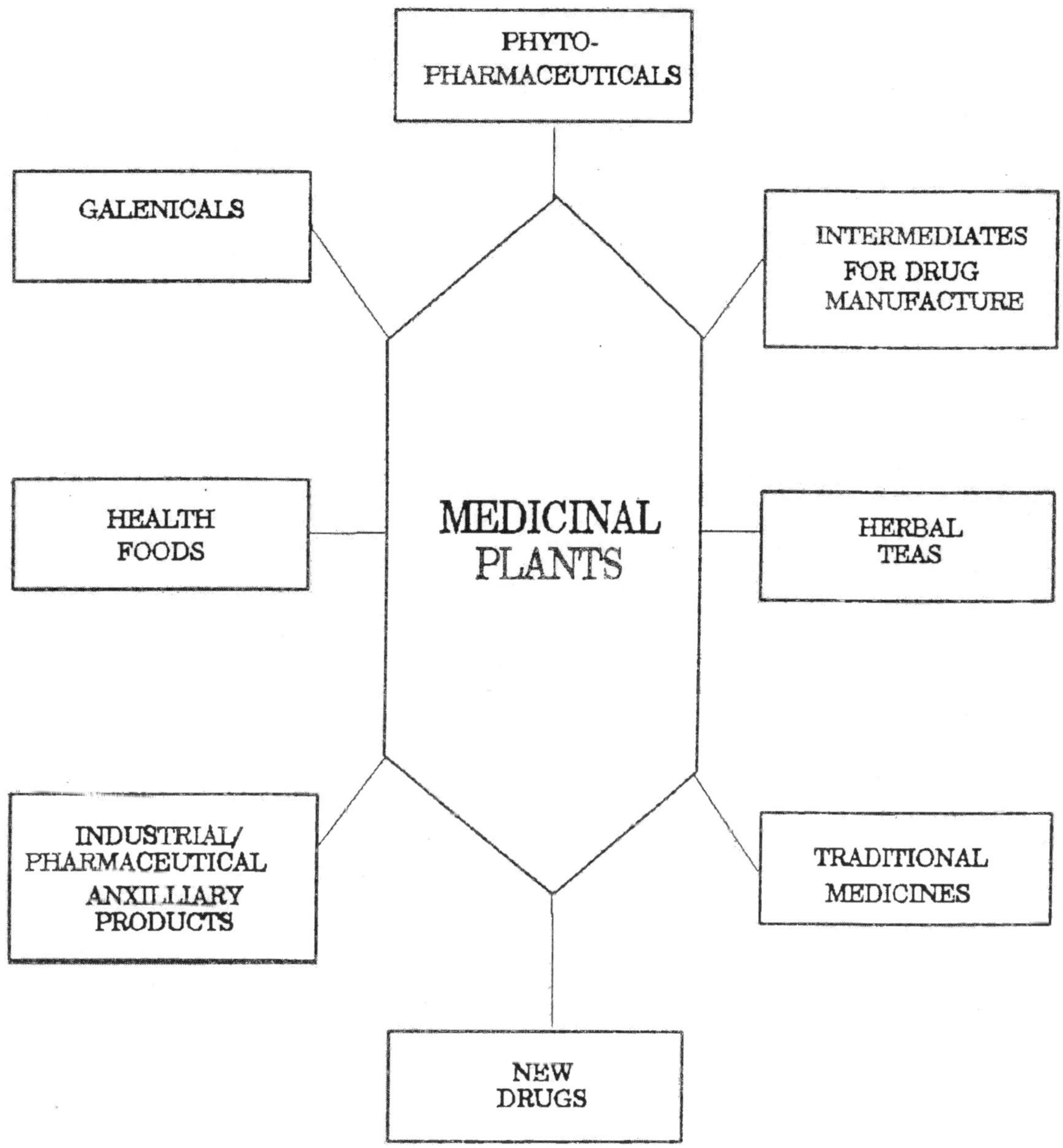

Figure 1: Industrial uses of Medicinal Plants

conservation of biodiversity through small-scale production and preservation of cultural knowledge. Use of sophisticated modern technology will alienate the traditional practitioner as he has no control over such production methods. Even in the use of appropriate technologies, the practitioner who produces these drugs has to be educated about the advantages of using such production and quality control methods.

One major concern in introducing modern technology for the production of traditional medicines is whether the final preparation will be acceptable to the practitioner who has sole faith in extemporaneous preparations. This problem has to be overcome by a process of education, whereby the disadvantages of the old methods and the advantages of the new methods can be imparted.

Value added products

The value of medicinal plants as a source of foreign exchange for developing countries depends on the use of those plants as raw materials in the pharmaceutical industry. These raw materials are used to:

- Isolate pure active compounds for formulation into drugs (quinine, reserpine,digoxin,etc.)
- Isolate intermediates for the production of semi-synthetic drugs
- Prepare standardised galenicals (extracts, powders, tinctures, etc.)

If one is to produce known pure phytopharmaceuticals used in modern medicine, more processing stages and more sophisticated machinery are required. Furthermore, safety and pollution aspects have to be considered. Most of these processes and formulations are patent-protected. Even transferring technology through contractual agreements and payment will not be of much help unless there is a large local demand for these drugs. Often the drugs so produced are more expensive than world market prices owing to the limitations of the economy of scale of production.

Certain plants are rich sources of intermediates used in the production of drugs. The primary processing of parts of plants containing the intermediates could be carried out in the country of origin thus retaining some value of the resource material. For example, diosgenin (from *Dioscorea* sp.) and hecogenin (from sisal) used in the production of steroids can be commercially produced in the countries of origin where there are steady supplies of sufficient raw materials.

Processed products (galenicals) from plants could be standardised fluid/solid extracts or powders or tinctures. Standardised extracts of many plants (e.g. *Aloe* species, *Atropa belladonna*, *Cassia angustifolia*, *Capsicum annuum*, *Centella asiatica*, *Cephaelis ipecacuanha*, *Digitalis* species, *Commiphora mukul*, *Panax ginseng*) are widely used in health care. Some of these have to be formulated for incorporation into modern dosage forms. New formulations require some development work, particularly on account of the nature of the processed products. Plant extracts are difficult to granulate, sensitive to moisture and prone to microbial contamination. Hence the types of excipients to be used and the processing parameters have to be determined.

Downstream processing activities leading to different medicinal plant based products are indicated in Figure. 2.

Most of the activities of UNIDO in the industrial utilization of medicinal plants have involved: the production of standardised traditional medicines, galenicals and extracts, the formulation and development of dosage forms, the development of new preparations based on the traditional pharmacopoeia, research and development in processing and formulation and basic chemical and pharmacological studies. Processing using clean and pollution free technologies have been introduced.

Pilot scale production

Development of process parameters has to be carried out at a pilot scale in order to be upscaled to industrial production. Many R&D institutions and universities in developing countries do not have such facilities and are therefore unable to pass on their R&D findings to the industry. UNIDO has played a significant role in achieving university-industry interaction by designing a polyvalent pilot plant which could be used for many unit operations needed for the production of plant-based products. Detailed engineering drawings with specifications and bills of quantities are published in a separate UNIDO publication (UNIDO, 1991). The pilot plant has enabled the R & D work to be demonstrated to produce final products which could be market tested. Universities in turn have been able to realize the hidden potential of industrialization of their R & D work. Any institution which wants to initiate downstream processing of medicinal plants and other non-wood forest products should possess facilities for pilot scale production.

New technologies

Improved methods for the processing of medicinal and aromatic plants and new techniques for quality assessment are being developed rapidly and continuously and they have to be introduced to developing countries if they are to forge ahead to keep up with recent developments and new international requirements. One such method of recent development is Supercritical Fluid Extraction of natural products as an alternative for solvent extraction. It is now used both for processing of phytopharmaceuticals and other plant products and for the removal of trace amounts of contaminant substances such as pesticides, toxins and surfactants.

Quality assurance

The control of the quality of the raw materials, finished products and of processes is an absolute necessity, if one is to produce goods for world markets and human consumption.

International Standard Specifications exist for some processed products and some countries and buyers have their own requirements. The quality requirements for medicinal plant preparations are stringent in terms of content of active principles and toxic materials. Whereas the production of traditional medicines for local use does not require such stringent standards, what is produced will be a much more improved version of the already produced medicines using traditional methods.

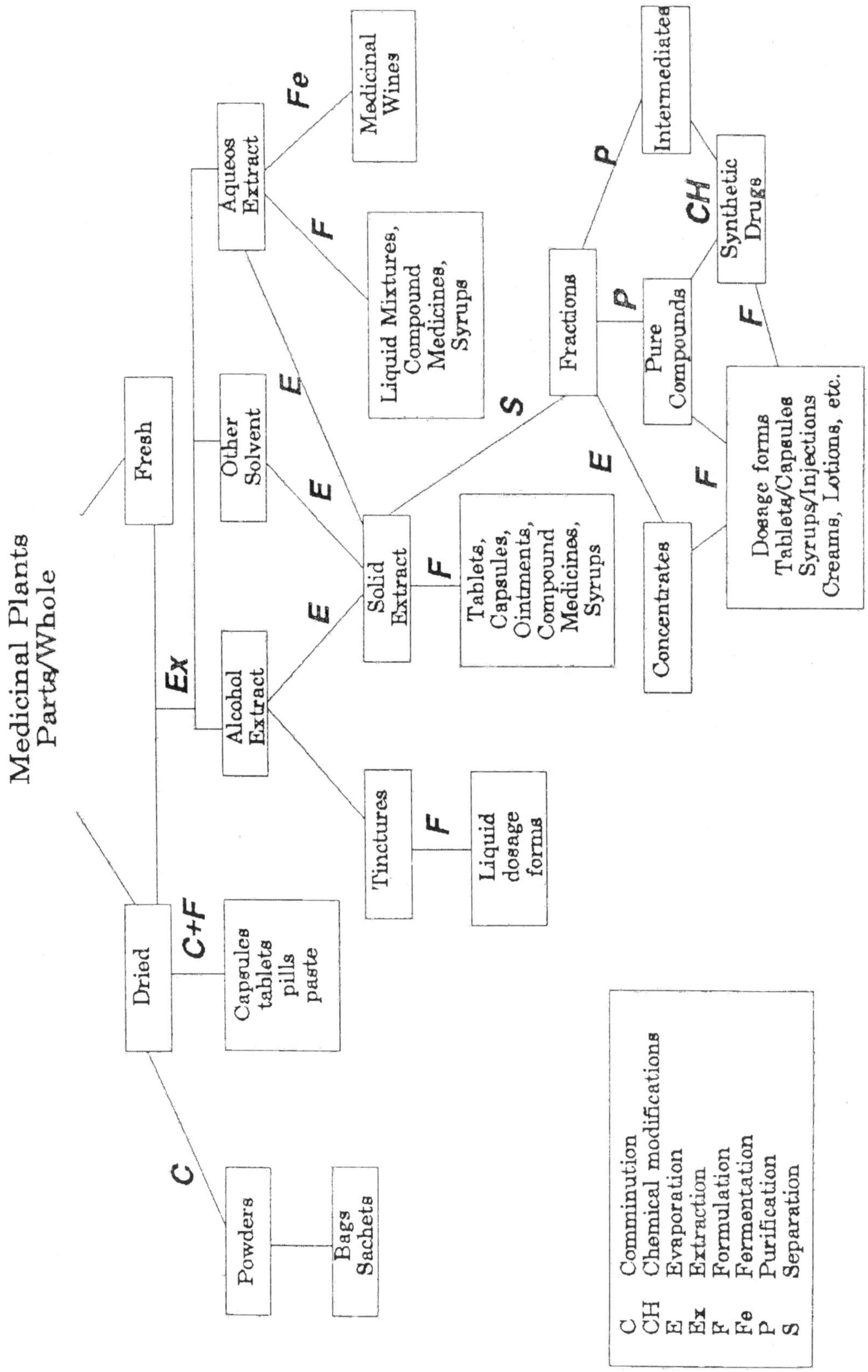

Figure 2: Downstream processes

Quality has to be built into the whole process beginning from the selection of propagation material to the final product reaching the consumer. It is therefore a management system where all steps involved in the industrial utilization process have to be properly and strictly controlled to produce the desired quality products. All elements of Total Quality Management(TQM) have to be introduced in any industrial project. The requirements for ISO 9000 certification and Good Manufacturing Practices(GMP) have to be introduced and the personnel trained so that enterprises could introduce the proper systems needed for certification. Furthermore eco-audit procedures (ISO 14000) leading to eco-labelling will be required for safeguarding environmental damage.

Human resource development

Many developing countries have a core of trained personnel in the fields of chemistry, biology, agriculture, pharmacology and pharmacy: They lack resources in such fields as chemical engineering and technology. This can be considered as a major constraint upon industrial development. UNIDO therefore has developed the human resources required for this specific area of industrial development by conducting training in industrial practice including quality assurance, management and marketing.

Marketing

Marketing is an unsurmountable problem besetting the development of the plant-based industry in developing countries and marketability will be a crucial factor in determining the failure or success of these industries. The market outlets can be for local use and for export. As for local use, some products could reach the consumer directly while others have to be either further processed or used as secondary components in other industrial products. Hence user industries have to be promoted so that locally produced extracts can be used to save foreign exchange needed for importation of such additives.

Further processing to yield value added products will be limited by the local demand situation unless they could be produced at prices to be competitive in the world market. Even if the cost of production is low and quality of the products is good, substantial market promotion has to be undertaken in order to penetrate the world market.

Market tie-ups with progressive entrepreneurs from the developed world would be a convenient and a realistic option for securing markets for the finished products. Joint ventures or trade agreements could be initiated with companies that are expanding their production to meet the ever increasing demand for green products.

Research and development

Industrial development requires parallel research and development. Research in chemistry and bioactive components of indigenous flora of developing countries has been ongoing for quite some time, funded by multi-/ bi- lateral aid or non-governmental donor organisations. A systematic and a concerted approach to this activity has not been maintained for want of sophisticated equipment and high-cost chemicals. Much of the research has been mainly academic. The concept of applied research in the industrial use of plants has not received much attention.

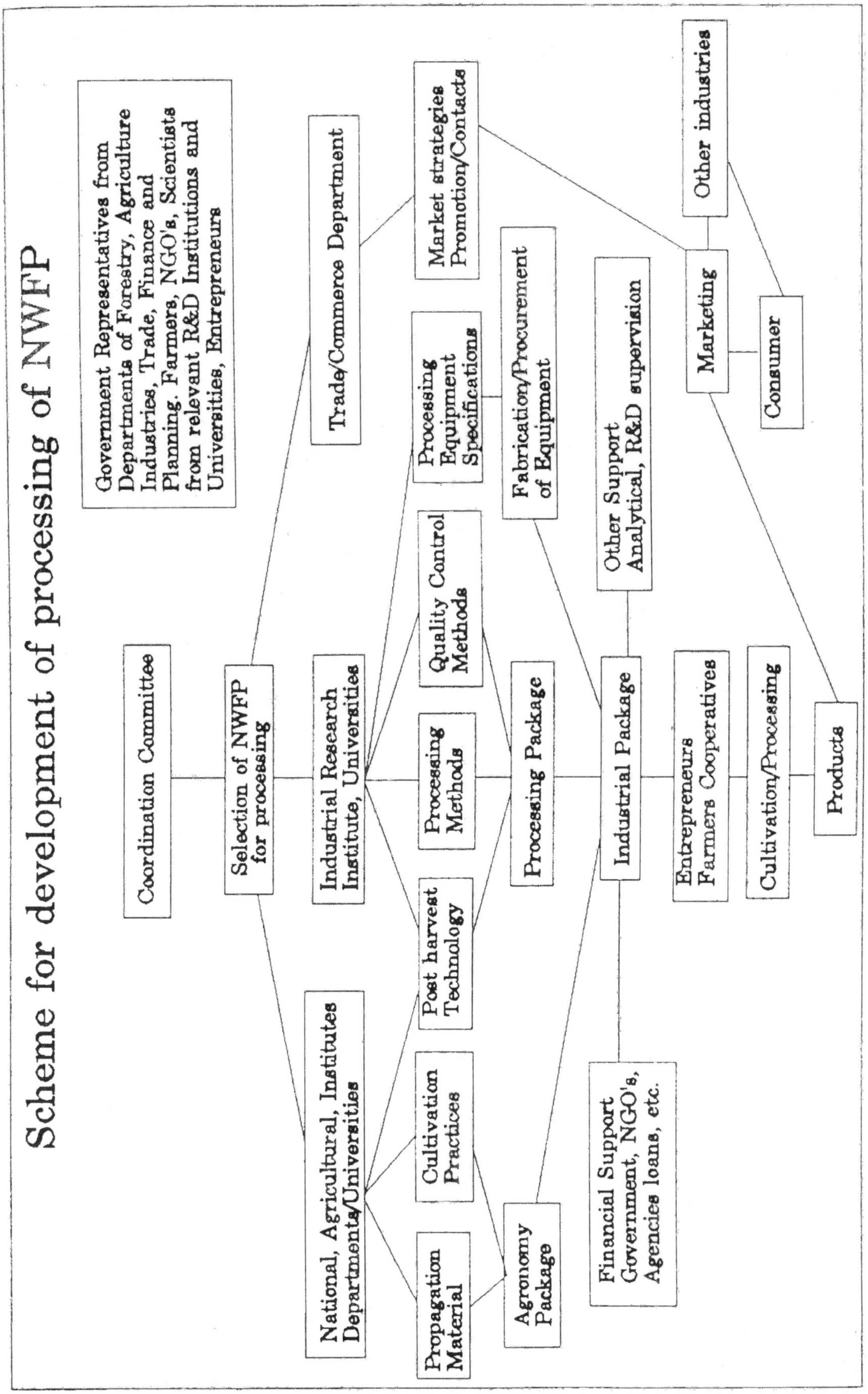

Figure 3: Scheme for development of processing of NWFP

Research in support of industrial development encompasses all activities ranging from the development of superior propagation materials, agrotechnology, low cost and efficient processing technologies to improve quality and yield, new formulations to new products and the marketing of finished products.

Registration and property rights

Many developing countries do not have procedures to register medicinal plant preparations although they are widely used for the health care needs of the majority of people. The regulations if any, are very stringent requiring the same standards expected of modern medicines. WHO has recently published guidelines for the assessment of herbal medicines taking into account the long and extensive usage of them (WHO, 1991). These guidelines should encourage developing countries to relax some of the current regulations to be realistic in recognizing the role of traditional medicines in the health care delivery of their countries.

The vital question of property rights to developing countries for the use of know-how and genetic resources in the development of modern drugs in developed countries has been discussed in many forums but without a final solution.

Technical information

As the use of plant-based drugs has declined with the introduction of synthetic drugs especially in developing countries, the need to collate all available knowledge on medicinal plants and their uses has become imperative particularly because of the recent revival of interest in the use of "natural" medicines. In view of the greater demand for information on traditional uses and proper identification, and the enormous volume of information being generated, a user-friendly information storage and retrieval system will be of considerable importance. As such a computer database would be of invaluable assistance to developing countries in R & D work on industrial utilization of local plant resources.

Data on the medicinal plants are also available in international journals and a number of databases, the premier being Napralert established at the University of Illinois in Chicago with WHO assistance. Many developing countries lack the resources to subscribe to research journals or acquire access to these databases. In fact, the data required by the scientific personnel in developing countries with respect to technologies and methods used for processing and formulation of medicinal plants are not readily available in the literature nor in the databases as some of these are patent-protected.

Conclusions

A scheme for the establishment of processing industries based on plants is given in Figure. 3. It must be emphasised that the proper coordination of the multidisciplinary activities needed for processing is vital for the success of industries venturing into this field.

The development of any industrial processing activity has to be linked to the specific needs, socio-cultural background, resource potential and the technological capabilities of each country. Consequently, any integrated development approach adopted has to exploit the full potential of this natural resource by providing a proper scientific, technological, economic and an industrial base. Above all, developing countries' research and development capabilities, including human resources, have to be greatly enhanced so as to ensure the growth of industries based on medicinal and aromatic plants.

Sustainable development of industries based on plants requires multi-disciplinary activities and close collaboration between scientists, government officials, NGOs and international organizations. Such efforts have not received much attention resulting in the slow development of the economic uses of renewable resources. Hence it is important that more action-oriented plans are initiated to exploit the full potential of these resources, bearing in mind the conservation issues such that rural household incomes and national economies could be augmented.

References

De Silva T. 1996. *A Manual on the Essential Oil Industry*. Vienna, Austria; United Nations Industrial Development Organisation. 232 pp.

De Silva, T. & Atal, C.K. 1995. *Processing, Refinement and Value Addition of Non-wood Forest Products*. FAO report of the International Expert Consultation on Non-wood Forest Products pp.167-193.

De Silva, T. 1993. UNIDO development programmes on industrial utilization of medicinal and aromatic plants. *Acta Horticulturae* 333: 47-54.

Tcheknavorian-Asenbauer, A. 1993. Industrial utilization of medicinal and aromatic plant resources in developing countries. *Acta Horticulturae* 333: 19-46.

Tcheknavorian-Asenbauer, A. *et al.* 1982. *Traditional Pharmacopoeia Revisited*. UNIDO IO.511.

Tcheknavorian-Asenbauer, A. & Wijesekera, R.O.B. 1982. *Industrial Utilization of Medicinal and Aromatic Plants*. UNIDO IO.505.

United Nations Industrial development Organization. 1991. *Design Options for a Polyvalent Pilot Plant Unit for the Distillation and Extraction of Medicinal and Aromatic Plants*.IPCT.143(spec).

Wijesekera, R.O.B. 1991. Is there an industrial future for phytopharmaceutical drugs? An outline of UNIDO programmes in the sector. *Journal of Ethnopharmacology* 32: 217-224.

Wijesekera, R.O.B. 1987. *Renaissance of the Phytopharmaca*. Vienna, Austria; United Nations Industrial Development Organization.

World Health Organization. 1991. *Guidelines for the Assessment of Herbal Medicines*. Geneva; Switzerland; WHO.

Trade in Medicinal Plants

Sophie Emma Kuipers
Natural Medicine Marketing
261 Portobello Road
W11 1LR London, UK
Tel/Fax: + +44 171 727 1753 Email: sophie@nat-med.demon.co.uk

Abstract

Medicinal plants play a critical role in the healthcare provision of much of the world's population. Whether they are used to make a decoction in rural Africa, to extract an alkaloid in Switzerland or as a health food supplement in the United States, demand is increasing. This paper attempts to examine the trade in medicinal plants; determine the volume of medicinal plant material that is traded and identify the main sources of demand and supply. In so doing the paper addresses the conservation implications arising from the trade and considers some possible solutions.

Medicinal plant demand

Before considering the sources of medicinal plants and mechanics of the trade, an understanding of where the demand for medicinal plants comes from is needed.

Medicinal plant material is used by a large number of industries. This paper attempts to focus mainly on demand from industries which use these plants for their medicinal or health giving properties as explained below. The problem lies in the fact that statistical data do not usually differentiate between these groups and other users such as manufacturers of: cosmetics, detergents, dyes, insecticides, foods, paints etc.

Pharmaceutical companies

This sector uses medicinal plants:

- for the isolation of single purified drugs, e.g. digitoxin extracted from digitalis and vincristine from *Catharanthus roseus*.

- in advanced extract form where the extract is highly standardised in terms of the active constituents it contains. In many cases, these are in admixtures with other ingredients, e.g. senna extract from *Cassia senna*.

- as starting material for the production of other semi-synthetic pharmacologically active substances. For example, plant saponins can be extracted and altered chemically to produce sapogenins required to manufacture steroids.

Demand for medicinal plants from this group alone is significant with an estimated 25% of prescription drugs in the US containing plant extracts or active principles prepared from higher plants (Farnsworth and Soejarto, 1985).

Phytopharmaceutical companies

In some countries (e.g. Germany), there is little distinction between pharmaceutical and phytopharmaceutical companies as both may sell products made from standardised extracts of plant material. However, in other countries where the licensing criteria for plant extracts are very different from those for medicines, there is more of a distinction.

Phytopharmaceutical companies not only use plant extracts but also raw plant material for example to make tinctures, teas or in capsule form.

Health product companies

Examples of some of the more important health products are garlic, ginseng, propolis, royal jelly, tonics, guarana and herbal drinks for which there has been a growing demand recently.

There is also a fine line of distinction between health products and phytopharmaceuticals as many health products are being marketed as such in order to avoid the need to license a product as a medicine (a costly and complex process).

Traditional medicines

Although traditional medicines could equally be covered under phytopharmaceuticals, a distinction is made here in order to highlight their importance in the medicinal plants trade. The WHO estimated that 80% of the population of developing countries rely on traditional medicines (primarily plant drugs) for their primary healthcare needs.

The most renowned traditional systems are Ayurvedic, Unani and traditional Chinese medicine (TCM). In addition, there are many less well documented systems of traditional medicine which have been handed down from one generation to the next by word of mouth and practised in many parts of the world. In the Côte d'Ivoire, a market survey of 800 households found that traditional medicines were not just used in rural areas but increasingly in urban areas as well (Bodeker, 1997).

Alternative practitioners

In addition to the traditional medicine practitioners in developing countries, there are an increasing number of alternative practitioners of natural medicine in the developed world.

Demand for medicinal plants is undoubtedly increasing in all the above sectors (with the possible exception of their use as pure chemical isolates) and this growth is fuelling an increase in both the number of species and volume of plant material being traded. What we now need to consider is from what sources this demand is being met.

Medicinal plant species

It is estimated that some 10,000 plant species are used medicinally, most of these are used in traditional systems of medicine. However, only a relatively small number of species are used in any significant volume. For example, in TCM, 9,905 botanical materials are used but only an estimated 500 are commonly used. (Natural Medicine Marketing, 1996).

A study undertaken by the International Trade Centre (ITC) in 1982 suggested that 400 species were used in Europe (ITC-UNCTAD GATT, 1982). More recent findings suggest that the number could be closer to 1,500 including those used in homeopathy (Lange, 1996). There are no reliable data on the number of plant species that are currently traded in high volume; indeed, such a list is badly needed.

An analysis of plant derived materials used in prescription drugs during 1980 found that only 40 species of higher plants are used as sources of drugs. (Farnsworth *et al.*, 1986).

Medicinal plant supply

There are two sources of supply of medicinal plants, *viz.* material collected from the wild and cultivated material. Surprisingly, the bulk of the material traded is still wild harvested and only a very small number of species is cultivated.

Wild harvested material

Wild harvesting is the collection of plant material such as the *herba* (plant above ground), *flos* (flowers), *folia* (leaves), *lignum* (wood), or *radix* (roots) from wild sources. In many traditions of medicine, wild harvested material is considered to have higher therapeutic benefits, and therefore, for example in China, commands higher prices.

Although there are many common species that can be harvested sustainably and with little impact on their survival, an increasing number are not in this category. A study undertaken by WWF found that in several African countries, wild harvesting for local requirements was not detrimental to plant survival as the quantity collected tended to be small and also most of the material collected came from the more common varieties (Hamilton, 1990).

What is of major concern is the fact that a major part of wild harvested material is now traded commercially. As the prices paid to the gatherers tend to be very low, commercial plant gatherers, often 'mine' the natural resources rather than manage them, as their main objective is to generate an income.

A critical factor in wild harvesting is the availability of cheap labour to undertake the very labour intensive work of gathering. As in many cases income from such sources represents the only form of paid employment for members of remote rural areas, there is an eagerness to undertake such work.

Most countries have little or no regulations controlling the collection of material from the wild. India is one exception and has banned the export of several wild species in the form of raw material although the export of finished products containing the material is allowed. Despite this, an estimated 95% of medicinal plants collected in India are gathered from the wild and the process of collection is said to be destructive (Vinay, 1996). Equally, a major part of the high range Himalayan plants are wild harvested and many of these are close to extinction from over-harvesting or unskilful harvesting e.g. *Nardostachys jatamansi*, *Aconitum* spp.

An estimated 70-90% of the medicinal plant material imported into Germany is wild harvested and only 50-100 species among these are currently propagated on a large scale (Lange, 1996).

In China, the output of the area cultivated is estimated to be between 300,000 and 400,000 tonnes whilst in 1994 the total demand for medicinal plant material was 1,600,000 tonnes. This huge gap must be made up from wild harvested material. What is particularly worrying is that TCM tends to use the roots of plants which are the most difficult plant parts to harvest sustainably.

Although the major part of wild harvested material is sourced from developing countries, a surprisingly high amount is also gathered in developed countries. For example, in the United States, an estimated 200 tons of *Echinacea angustifolia* is wild harvested annually (Foster, 1994) and 220,589 pounds of ginseng was wild harvested in 1992 (Gaski and Johnson). In France, more than 500 species were wild harvested during 1988-89, including those used homeopathically, i.e. in minute quantities. Volumes harvested for the most important among these are listed in Table 1.

Table 1. Tonnage of wild harvested material for leading medicinal plants in France during 1988-89 (adapted from Rolland, 1991).

Plant species	**Tonnage of dried plant material**
Arnica montana	3-6
Betula pendula& Betula pubescens	5-10
Calluna vulgaris	50
Conyza canadensis	50
Fraxinus excelsior	50
Hippophae rhamnoides	5-10
Hypericum perforatum	50-100
Prunus spinosa	5-10
Rhamnus frangula	5-10
Rosmarinus officinalis	50-100
Ruscus aculeatus	5-10
Sorbus aucuparia	50
Filipendula ulmaria	5-10

Although one can cite data for some such specific cases, there is very little global data on the volume wild harvested. This is partly because it is very difficult to distinguish between wild and cultivated material, as such wild harvested material is often sold as cultivated. This means that even CITES (Convention on International Trade in Endangered

Species) data are often questionable given that the process of issuing licenses and acquiring import/export papers as required by CITES is rarely checked and may often be the subject of corruption.

Cultivation

The other main source of medicinal plants is from cultivation. Cultivated material is infinitely more appropriate for use in the production of drugs. Indeed, standardisation whether for pure products, extracts or crude drugs is critical, and will become increasingly so, as quality requirements continue to become more stringent.

Examples of countries that do cultivate on a large scale are Hungary, Poland, India (psyllium), China, Spain (liquorice), and Argentina (chamomile, psyllium). Requirements of successful commercial cultivation operations are to produce high quality drugs using low input cultivation methods keeping in mind that the material has to compete within a highly competitive international market.

Given the higher cost of cultivated material, cultivation is often done under contract. In the majority of cases, companies would cultivate only those plant species which they use in large quantities or in the production of derivatives and isolates, for which standardisation is essential and quality is critical.

More recently, growers have set up co-operatives or collaborative ventures in an attempt to improve their negotiating power and achieve higher prices. One such co-operative is VNK in the Netherlands; others have also emerged in Eastern Europe to help them compete in a now privatised sector. Eastern Europe exports significant quantities to the rest of Europe and North America. Before the subsidies were cancelled post-1989, these countries were reliable suppliers of good quality material. However, since then reliability and quality have become a problem.

The question that begs to be asked is why more material is not cultivated internationally. There are several reasons, notably the low cost of wild harvested material, and the fact that cultivated material requires management/agricultural expertise, time (sometimes more than 10 years before the crop is ready for harvesting), land, financial resources etc. before an income can be derived.

Channels of supply

The following section considers the different forms of trade that exist and examines the channels through which medicinal plants pass.

Cunningham (1996) describes three trading sectors for medicinal plants:

- On the first level, there is the national trade in medicinal plants which can involve hundreds of species. This trade would be undertaken at regional medicinal plant markets where hundreds of plant species are traded. For example in urban markets in Kwa Zulu, Natal, more than 400 species were being traded out of a total 1,000 that were used medicinally in the area.

- The second level again is informal and consists of trade across national borders but within the same continent. This trade tends to consist of fewer number of species, although many of these are threatened. For example in Africa, *Warburgia salutaris* and *Siphonochilus aethiopicus* are two species with high demand and very scarce supply. In Asia, *Nardostachys grandiflora* and *Valeriana jatamansi* are examples of species which are threatened, but both are still traded from Nepal to India (Cunningham, 1996).

- The third level comprises formal export trade. In Africa, Cunningham found that at this level only a limited number of species were traded in significant volumes. Cunningham cites Cameroon which exports four species to Europe including *Prunus africana* (a bark extract of which is used in the treatment of benign prostatic hypertrophy), all of which is exported to France; and *Pausinystalia johimbe*, 65% of which is exported to Holland, 18% to Germany and the rest to Belgium, Luxembourg and France.

However, based on the imports of plant material into Germany, a significant number of species are indeed traded internationally, i.e. at this third level, and several hundred species in significant volumes.

From the source of collection, plant material passes through a network of buyers including collectives' organisations and state run organisations, and agents or subsidiaries of the plant traders.

The major part of material is sold to plant trading companies. These plant traders hold enormous stocks, and also have the facilities to undertake the quality controls required for raw material used in the production of drugs. The major trading companies are located in Hamburg, New York, Tokyo and Hong Kong. They play an enormously powerful role in the medicinal plant trade, partly because of the large quantities they purchase which enables them to more or less dictate the price. In addition, their ability to reliably undertake the quality control analysis also helps to protect their position of power.

The situation in Germany illustrates the critical role of the traders, where 'drug' imports of medicinal plants is undertaken almost entirely by 20 drug trading companies (Lange, 1996).

Another critical point which helps safeguard the position of the traders is the guarantee that they will supply material of a specified standard of quality at a fixed price. This price and quality guarantee is a major incentive to the end user, for whom cost, quality, reliability and flexibility are said to be the key requirements for purchasing pharmaceutical raw materials (Lapinskas, 1993).

There are also brokers who buy plant material and sell it on adding a commission; however, they do not stock material or have any warehousing facilities. In the past the brokers played a more important role as they had the contacts at the purchasing level.

Other traders have been emerging, referred to as the 'ecological trade' by Lange (1996), they source botanical material for use generally by the smaller herbal medicine/health product companies and alternative practitioners. These trading companies tend to be more discerning/ethical in their purchasing approach, and often trade extensively in organically cultivated products. They often establish their own contacts in the source countries and have shorter sales routes involving fewer parties, partly as they purchase only raw material not extracts.

One such example is a company in the United Kingdom called Hambledon Herbs (HH), who endeavour to build relationships with trustworthy and ethical suppliers who practise sustainable harvesting or organic/semi-organic cultivation methods. For example, Hambledon Herbs source *Harpagophytum* from Namibia as part of a conservation project that they have set up with Oxfam. The material is collected from the wild in a controlled and sustainable way, planting is encouraged, and quality control measures have been introduced. HH are now the leading supplier of *Harpagophytum,* supplying an estimated 50 tonnes per annum.

Plant extracts

A significant percentage of medicinal plant material is used to make plant extracts. This process is carried out either by the end product manufacturers or by extract companies. Sales of plant extracts is undoubtedly increasing as evidenced by the growth of one of Europe's leading extract suppliers, Indena, which increased its operating revenue by 92% from 1991 to 1994 (according to F&S Database compiled by Frost and Sullivan Publishers, London).

More recently, several extract companies have been set up in the Far East, in an attempt to increase the value of the raw material through processing. For example, Qingdao Huanzhong Pharmaceutical Ltd is a Sino-Japanese joint venture in China with a production capacity of 240 tonnes of extracts all of which is destined for export to Japan and other international markets. Another example is that of Southern Herbals in India which started production in 1992 of plant extracts and is reported to be supplying companies such as Amgen, Bristol-Myers Squibb and Fujisawa with vincristine and vinblastine from *Catharanthus roseus*.

Volume traded

Having examined the channels of supply, consideration needs to be given to the volume that passes through those channels. Unfortunately, there are very few data on the volume of international trade in medicinal plants. What little data there are, are further complicated by the fact that medicinal plants are, as previously mentioned, used in many other industries.

Much of the following data have been sourced from the UNCTAD COMTRADE database and compiled from statistical information from approximately 100 countries. The other main source of data is the market report published by the German Federal Agency for Nature Conservation (Lange, 1996). With both sources, the SITC codes used to compile the data (Table 2) need to be considered in the light of the fact that they are not exclusively used as medicinal plants.

Table 2. SITC codes and Commodity codes.

SITC code		Commodity code
292.4	Plants and parts of plants (including seeds and fruit) of a kind used primarily in perfumery, in pharmacy, or for insecticidal, fungicidal, or similar purposes	140190 00 0
292.41	Liquorice roots	1211.10
292.42	Ginseng roots	1211.20
292.49	Others including pyrethrum, tonquin beds, mint, linden, verbena, *Origanum vulgare* and *Salvia officinalis*	1211.90

Furthermore, the data do not include the trade in glycosides and vegetable alkaloid derivatives which are both important raw materials to the pharmaceutical industry. Table 3 provides some perspective on the growth in sales of glycosides and vegetable alkaloids based on the increased quantities being imported globally.

Table 3. Global imports of vegetable alkaloids, glycosides and their derivatives.

Year	Imports of vegetable alkaloids and derivatives Standard units in Million kg	Imports of glycosides and derivatives Standard units in Million kg
1966	1,922,449	312,252
1976	4,339,750	621,569
1986	13,359,933	1,984,916
1988	13,839,193	2,524,890
1990	12,516,068	3,016,647
1991	11,412,323	2,929,112

Source: United Nations Statistical Division (1992)

Major supplying countries and regions

This section seeks to identify the major source countries for medicinal plants traded internationally.

The main geographical areas supplying medicinal plants to Germany are listed in Table 4 which provides an understanding of the source of material used in Europe and North America.

Table 4: Quantity of imports of commodity groups 1211 90 80 and 1211 90 90(0) [Plants and parts of seeds...-others] classified according to areas of origin (adapted from Lange, 1996).

Volume tonnes	1994	1993	1992	1991
Europe (incl. regions of the former USSR)	14,062.9	11,932.4	16,578.6	14,799.2
Asia	7,708.1	7,518.1	9,080.3	9,487.3
Africa	7,374.8	6,047.7	4,949.6	4,642.4
America	5,065.0	6,258.4	7,705.5	5,257.1
Australia & New Zealand	416,5	419.3	530.4	651.7
Others	734.9	129.8	106.7	69.6

Table 5 provides more information on which countries in each geographical region, are important suppliers of raw material to Germany (indicative of trends in exports to Europe and North America).

Table 6 gives more of an international perspective in that it identifies the leading exporters of medicinal plant material in general, i.e. not to any specific market. Again these data highlight the importance of Asia as a supplier of medicinal plants.

Table 5. Countries with exports to Germany in excess of 500 tonnes for Commodity Codes 1211 90 80bzw 1211 90 90 (0) (adapted from Lange, 1996). Volume exported to Germany in tonnes.

Country	1994	1993	1992	1991
EUROPE				
France	1,011.4	1,016.7	748.7	670.0
Netherlands	641.6			684.5
Greece			580.9	601.5
Austria	1,125.3	1,169.9	1,247.6	
Yugoslavia				1,457.6
Croatia	557.8			
Poland	2,065.8	2,168.3	2,142.8	2,209.2
Hungary	2,185.0	2,039.5	2,170.2	1,623.5
Rumania	656.9		747.5	
Bulgaria	2,723.3	1,360.1	3,487.6	3,644.3
Albania	1,471.4	1,158.7	2,296.9	1,876.2
ASIA				
Turkey	608.4	500.1	1,208.4	990.1
India	4,247.3	4,294.3	3,981.3	6,040.1
Thailand		651.1	1,236.9	
China	1,594.6	1,336.7	1,633.3	1,420.5
AFRICA				
Morocco			567.8	562.5
Egypt	1,729.1	1,351.2	1,687.0	1,987.0
Sudan	3,755.4	2,891.4	1,949.1	1,655.8
Zaire	912.1	728.4		
AMERICA				
USA	1,172.7	789.3	1,767.3	1,119.8
Brazil		658.8	670.0	579.2
Chile	1,711.3	2,440.6	2,934.4	961.7
Argentina	1,129.0	1,477.2	1,812.9	2,204.5
OTHERS				
Australia			530.4	648.2
Anonymous countries	535.7	522.5	899.3	952.0
TOTAL	35,362.1	32,832.5	42,346.7	35,849.1

Table 6. Leading exporters of PHARMACH PLANTES NES (sitc. 3 29249 cccn:1211): value in in excess of US$ 10,000,000.

COUNTRY	Unit US$ 000 1995	INDEX 1995/1991
SUM WORLD	879,757	136
China	337,162	204
Germany	49,887	89
USA, Puerto Rico, US Virgin Islands	36,269	146
France	23,505	84
OTH ASIA NES	23,148	84
Korea Rep.	20,125	112
Bulgaria	16,049	111
Italy	15,865	125
Thailand	15,806	100
Vietnam	15,237	283
Egypt	13,789	109
Hong Kong	12,767	103
Chile	10,582	239
Morocco	10,558	89
Albania	10,036	102

Major importing countries and regions

Germany

Germany dominates the European trade in medicinal plants as it dominates the European market for phytopharmaceuticals. During the last three years, 40,000 tonnes of 'botanicals' were imported annually into Germany with a value of US$ 109 million (DM 160 million) (Lange, 1996). These were from a total of 109 countries and one-third of the material was re-exported as finished plant based products primarily to Western Europe and the United States.

North America

North America is another important importing region for medicinal plant material. IUCN/WWF sources estimate the annual turnover of the plant derived pharmaceuticals industry in the US at US$ 10 billion (IUCN-WWF, 1988). Retail sales of the herbal medicines industry in 1994 were estimated at US$ 1.6 billion. Indeed, the North American health products market is a fast growing market and its demand for medicinal plant material is significant. The major part of material is sourced from Europe (notably Eastern Europe) and Asia. Over the last five years, demand in North America for Latin American herbs and Chinese and Indian material has also been significant.

Asia

The major importers of medicinal plants in Asia are Hong Kong (most of its imports being destined for mainland China), and Japan.

Traditional systems of medicine

When considering major sources of demand, the volumes of material used in traditional systems of medicine, particularly in Asia, need to be taken into account.

China's total output of medicinal plants from both cultivated and wild harvested sources is 1,600,000 tonnes. In comparison, that of Germany is relatively small at 40,000 tonnes. China is also a significant exporter of medicinal materials with export sales in 1993 reported as US$ 270 million although this figure does not only include plant material but also animal and mineral matter (Natural Medicine Marketing, 1996).

Ayurvedic and Unani herbs are also traded in large quantities and over a very wide geographical area. For example in 1992, an estimated 4,117,254 kg were exported, largely to Bangladesh, Japan, Pakistan, Saudi Arabia, USA and the UAE.

As already noted above, the major importers of medicinal plant material are Germany, China (via Hong Kong and Singapore) and Japan. The data presented in Table 7 substantiate this and identify other leading importers.

Table 7. Leading importers of PHARMACH PLANTES NES (sitc. 3 29249 cccn:1211): value in excess of US$ 10,000,000

COUNTRY	Unit US$ '000 1994	INDEX 1995/1991
SUM WORLD	824,212	227
Hong Kong	125,277	1,092
Germany	86,496	166
Japan	73,927	328
Singapore	60,519	729
OTH, ASIA NES	57,004	232
Korea Rep.	49,884	2,219
France	49,748	206
USA, PR, US VI	47,787	110
Malaysia	36,068	244
Italy	22,629	140
Switzerland	17,649	144
United Kingdom	17,504	150
Spain	15,636	121
Saudi Arabia	15,314	192
United ArabE	12,572	237
Canada	12,507	147
Belgium/Luxembourg	11,396	100
Netherlands	11,104	108

Conservation implications of medicinal plant trade

It is evident that the trade in medicinal plants has serious implications on the survival of some plant species. If one considers that 70-90% of material imported into Germany and 75% of material collected in China are wild harvested, the survival of some of these species may well be under threat, given the increasing demand for medicinal plants.

Although there are only a relatively small number of species that are traded in any significant volume, the fact that so few species (50-100) (Lange, 1996) are produced entirely under cultivation is a matter of great concern. Examples of major cultivated species are: *Catharanthus roseus*, *Chamomilla recutita*, *Cinchona* spp., *Digitalis lanata*, *D. purpurea*, *Duboisia* spp., *Mentha piperita*, *Papaver somniferum* and *Plantago ovata* (Lewington, 1993).

There are a number of reasons as to why the trade in wild harvested material has been left to reach such a critical point:

- Firstly, the legislation that exists to control harvesting and trade of medicinal plants is inadequate and ineffective in its current form; new policies and easier mechanisms to control the trade are needed.

- Secondly, the lack of awareness among many of the end users, as to the extent to which wild harvested materials are used; indeed, it is only during the last five to ten years that wild harvesting has become a subject of concern.

- Thirdly, in an attempt to control the market, the traders will give virtually no information on the extent of wild-harvesting.

- Finally, as already mentioned, the low price of wild harvested material has made the procurements of alternative sources of raw material (via cultivation) financially unattractive.

International policy and regulation

Despite the seriousness of the problem, there exist a limited number of measures for controlling international trade in medicinal plants. Currently the main form of regulation is through CITES (Convention on International Trade in Endangered Species of Wild Fauna and Flora). However, this agreement is not specifically concerned with medicinal plants and, in fact, has only a limited number of medicinal plants listed in the Appendices.

The CITES treaty was signed in Washington in 1973, and has signatories from 99 countries. The treaty functions on the basis of its three appendices, each of which sets out different trade restrictions (with no trade allowed for species listed under Appendix I). Only very recently has a list been compiled of medicinal plants that are included in CITES and only for plants that are in trade in Germany. Included in this list are 43 species. All except two are under Appendix 1 (more information on CITES, including the lists of species on the three appendices, can be downloaded from:http://www.unep.ch/cites.html).

New policy is needed and an easier mechanism to control the trade of plants. Apart from the recent (and continuing) involvement of The World Bank, most of the current conservation efforts seem to be led by non-governmental organisations and privately funded international agencies, notably World Conservation Monitoring Centre (WCMC), the Worldwide Fund for Nature (WWF), the Nature Conservancy (of USA), the World Conservation Union (IUCN), several botanic gardens, mainly Kew, Edinburgh, Missouri and New York.

The problem lies in the fact that there is little or no legislation restricting the use of wild-harvested materials in **finished** products, or for assuring the sustainable utilisation of medicinal plants.

The World Bank in its document 'Medicinal Plants; A Growing Role in Development' (Srivastava *et al.*, 1995) suggests that any national strategy for medicinal plant development needs to consider the following:

- 'Is the use of medicinal plants encouraged in healthcare programmes?
- Are there policies for conserving medicinal plants and incentives to encourage local community participation?
- Is there a policy for restoring plants harvested in the wild?
- Are there incentives for collectors and farmers to keep the production of medicinal plants sustainable?
- Does the Government support research into these plants?
- What are the policies regarding the export of medicinal plants?
- Are only raw materials exported?
- Is "in-country" processing (which may further help the trade in medicinal plants) being promoted? '

This same paper highlights the need for greater awareness of the issues particularly among government officials, farmers and scientists. It is also very obvious that there needs to be greater awareness amongst the end users, e.g. the pharmaceutical, phytopharmaceutical and health products companies, as to the consequences of their trade on the future availability of medicinal plant resources.

Dr Dagmar Lange suggests a combined approach where an attempt is made to encourage greater responsibility from not only the plant trading companies but also the end user companies and the consumers. Collective consumer pressure is a powerful tool in bringing about change in commercial practices. As such, consumers should be made aware of the problems with the medicinal plant trade and encouraged to only purchase products made from plants cultivated or collected on a sustainable basis. Perhaps an international logo similar to those used for recycled goods or for organically farmed foods can be used.

Although the problem of wild harvesting is of international concern, perhaps the developed world should first try to reduce the demand for such material.

References

Bodeker, G.C. 1997. Wound healing, traditional treatments and research policy. In: Houghton, P.(ed) *Modern Medicine and Traditional Remedies*. London, UK; Royal Pharmaceutical Society (in press).

Cunningham, A.B. 1996. Medicinal plant trade, conservation and the MPSG (Medicinal Plant Specialist Group) *Medicinal Plant Conservation* 2: 2-3.

Farnsworth, N.R.& Soejarto, D.D. 1985. Potential consequence of plant extinction in the United States on the current and future availability of prescription drugs. *Economic Botany* 39: (3) 231-240.

Farnsworth, N.R., Soejarto, D.D.& Bingel, A.S. 1986. Medicinal plants in therapy. *Bulletin of the World Health Organization* 63: (6) 965-981.

Foster, S. 1994. Commercial herb production: Conservation by cultivation. *Herbalgram* 32: 38.

Gaski, & Johnson, 'Prescription for Extinction' World Wildlife Foundation

Hamilton, A. 1990. La Conservation des plantes médicinales et autres végétaux utiles. *Bulletin de la Société Industrielle de Mulhouse.* No 819. pp 19-24.

ITC - UNCTAD GATT. 1982 *Markets for Selected Medicinal Plants and Their Derivatives*. Geneva, Switzerland; International Trade Center.

IUCN-WWF. 1988. Biodiversity: the Key to role for Plants. Kew, pp 7.

Lange, D. 1996. *Untersuchungen zum Heilpflanzenhandel in Deutschland.* Bonn, Germany; Bundesamt fur Naturschutz.

Lapinskas, P. 1993. Factors affecting the commercial success of a novel crop. *Acta Horticulturae* 333: 73-79.

Lewington, A. 1993. *A Review of the Importation of Medicinal Plants and Plant Extracts into Europe*. Cambridge, UK; TRAFFIC International. 37 pp.

Natural Medicine Marketing. 1996. *Market Report - Traditional Chinese Medicine - the Chinese Market and International Opportunities.* London, UK; Natural Medicine Marketing.

Rolland, A. 1991. Qualité des plantes médicinales, interêt et utilité des fiches de spécification. *Le Devenir des Plantes Utiles.* No 819. pp. 39-44.

Srivastava, J., Lambert, J.& Vietmeyer, N. 1995. *Medicinal Plants: A Growing Role in Development.* Washington, D.C., USA; Agricultural and Natural Resources Department, The World Bank.

UN Statistical Division. 1992.

Vinay, T. 1996.Camp workshop: Plants under threat - New list forged' *Medicinal Plant Conservation* Volume 2. Newsletter of the IUCN Species Survival Commission. Bonn, Germany; Bundesamt für Naturschutz.

Medicinal plant information databases

K. K. S. Bhat
Global Initiative For Traditional Systems (GIFTS) of Health,
Health Services Research Unit
Institute of Health Sciences, University of Oxford, UK
fax: + +44 1865 226711 Email: sbhat@medplant.demon.co.uk

Abstract

Information relating to medicinal plants can be found in documents and databases aimed at readers in a wide range of disciplines including botany, horticulture, chemistry, medicine, veterinary science, social sciences and economics. Recent developments in information technology and telecommunications have led to an increasing proportion of this literature now being available in electronic form. The range of primary, secondary and tertiary electronic publications available is reviewed and the contents of the main online databases and offline electronic products containing information on medicinal plants are described.

Introduction

Concomitant with the growing interest world-wide in the conservation, cultivation and use of medicinal, aromatic and other related groups of plants, there has been a four-fold increase in the volume of literature published on these plants during the past two decades (Bhat, 1995). Until early 1970s, printed publications were the almost exclusive means available for recording and disseminating scientific information. Developments in information technology during the 1980s and 1990s have led to an increasing proportion of this pool of information now being held in electronic form in databases which can either be searched online from remote sites or consulted offline at the reader's own desk.

Whereas the bulk of the information held in databases is still copied from or entered simultaneously with its appearance in printed publications, we are now beginning to see documents which are published exclusively in electronic form. Recent developments in telecommunications and information technology and the rapidly growing popularity of Internet as the medium of communication of the 1990s suggest that a significant proportion of information dissemination will occur through this medium within the next few years. Internet resources containing information on medicinal plants which cannot be found elsewhere have already started to appear. However, the present paper is mainly concerned with electronic databases providing information on medicinal plants which can be searched without being connected to the Internet.

Sources of information on medicinal plants

A. Primary publications

These are documents reporting current work or reviewing and analysing recent advances in knowledge. Documents in this category include journals reporting the results of original research, conference proceedings, annual and other reports published by various organisations, books, theses and patents. By far the most important among these are the primary journals. A recent survey (Bhat, 1995) involving extensive scanning of primary publications has shown that approximately a quarter of the total volume of literature currently being generated on medicinal and related groups of plants appears in less than ten periodicals. Approximately 50% of the total volume is contained in some 50 titles. However, the remaining 50% of this literature is scattered across some 2,500 periodicals in a wide range of disciplines.

Whereas the bulk of these documents constituting primary sources of information are still published in printed form, an increasing number of books, periodicals and reports are now also being made available in electronic form. Early developments in this area are typified by the weekly updated ADONIS CD-ROM launched a few years ago, which now delivers PDF and TIFF images of articles appearing in over 800 biomedical journals published by 80 European and North American publishers. More recently, ADONIS has been complemented by ExtraMED, the WHO-sponsored CD-ROM publication containing the text and illustrations of papers from over 290 medical journals published in developing countries (India, Pakistan, China, Philippines, Hong Kong, Korea, Singapore, Tanzania and Saudi Arabia among others). As might be expected, ExtraMED provides better coverage of literature in areas such as traditional medicine, tropical medicine, AIDS and waterborne diseases than ADONIS. Over the past year or so, some primary publications have also become available on the Internet.

B. Secondary and tertiary publications

Documents in this category are compiled from information previously published in primary source documents or that which is already common knowledge. They provide information in a summarised, 'digested', or otherwise 'processed' form rather than acting as vehicles for reporting new knowledge. They include various printed and electronic products derived from major bibliographic databases, abstracting and indexing periodicals, current awareness services, annotated bibliographies on specific topics, annual reviews and other books and periodicals which are dedicated to reviewing progress in specific areas, dictionaries, encyclopaedias, compendia, pharmacopoeias, directories, manuals and other reference works.

Compared with primary publications, a much greater proportion of secondary publications are available in electronic form. Many printed documents in this category are derived from data held in databases in electronic form.

Electronic databases

These may be classified into (a) secondary information databases (e.g. bibliographic databases) which give summaries of individual papers contained in primary publications and point the user to the original publication for further information; and (b) tertiary information databases (e.g. electronic compendia, encyclopaedias and other reference works) which give detailed information on specific topics and which may or may not indicate the source literature from which they are compiled.

The main differences between secondary and tertiary information databases are given in Table 1.

Table 1. A comparison of main features of secondary and tertiary information databases.

Secondary information database	Tertiary Information database
contents of each paper from primary publications are summarised by the abstractor/indexer	assembled by the compiler using information gathered selectively from a number of relevant sources
only contains previously published information	may contain information from unpublished sources
usually contains only views expressed by the author of the original paper	may contain compiler's own comments, observations etc.
each 'record' consists of full bibliographic details and an abstract of a single paper or document	each 'record' consists of encyclopaedic type of information on a specific topic or a sub-file containing a set of data contributing the compendium
usually (but with a few notable exceptions, e.g. patent abstract databases) provides information in textual form only	often contain illustrations, line diagrams, photographs, structural formulae etc. in addition to text
in-depth indexing using descriptors for organisms and concepts covered in the paper and subject classification to facilitate retrieval of information	subject indexing usually (but not necessarily) restricted to a limited number of keywords
updated at regular and frequent intervals by adding new records rather than by altering existing records	updated at infrequent intervals mainly by revising existing records to include new information.

Secondary information databases

Information on medicinal and other related groups of plants (which include herbs, spices and condiments; essential oil plants; plants containing compounds exhibiting insecticidal, molluscicidal, piscicidal, antifungal, antibacterial, antiviral or other biocidal activities; and poisonous plants) can be found in bibliographic databases dedicated exclusively to these groups of plants as well as in botanical, biological, agricultural, chemical, medical, veterinary or multidisciplinary databases with much wider subject coverage. The most important among these are listed below. Some of the secondary information databases published by organisations which also produce other types of publications are included in the section on tertiary information databases.

MAPA

Medicinal and Aromatic Plants Abstracts (MAPA) published by the National Institute of Science Communication (NISCOM, formerly known as the Publications and Information Directorate, Council of Scientific and Industrial Research), New Delhi, is a bimonthly printed journal in its 19th volume year. It provides good coverage of global literature on medicinal and aromatic plants. Over 55,000 abstracts have been published in the first 18 volumes of MAPA covering the period 1979-1996. The data from 1988 onwards (about 30,000 records) are also held in electronic form in the MAPA database and distributed on CD-ROM and other electronic media. Source literature currently scanned for compiling the database includes some 600 periodicals (of which about 200 are Indian) originating from 60 countries and published in 30 different languages. Conference proceedings, books and patents are also covered. Coverage of Indian and South-East Asian literature is particularly good and some records in this database are unique and cannot be found in other databases.

Contact: National Institute of Science Communication, Dr. K.S. Krishnan Road, New Delhi-110012, India. Telephone: (011) 574 6024; Fax: (011) 578 7062; Telex: 031-7721; E-mail: pid@sirnetd.ernet.in

CAB ABSTRACTS

Among multidisciplinary bibliographic databases, CAB ABSTRACTS provides the best all round coverage of world literature on medicinal and related groups of plants. Source literature scanned includes books, reports, conference proceedings and over 12,000 serials published from all over the world in a wide range of languages and covering virtually every discipline involved in the study of medicinal and related plants (botany, agronomy, biotechnology, phytochemistry, economics, medicine and veterinary science). Current rate of input of new material is over 150,000 records per year.

The database contains over 3 million bibliographic records prepared since 1972, of which approximately 60,000 are concerned with studies on medicinal and related groups of plants. The printed abstract journal, *Review of Aromatic and Medicinal Plants*, which is in its third volume year, provides excellent coverage of this literature. Earlier literature, dating back from 1931, which is not included in the electronic database, can be found in long-established CABI printed journals including *Horticultural Abstracts* and *Forest Products Abstracts*. These are among some 45 printed abstract journals published by CABI in the different disciplines covered in the database.

The database is made available to users through online and CD-ROM vendors such as DIALOG, DIMDI, ESA IRS, CAN-OLE, SILVER PLATTER, etc.

Contact: Marketing Department, CAB International, Wallingford, Oxon OX10 8DE, UK. Telephone: +44 1491 832111; Fax. +44 1491 833508; Telex: 847964 (COMAGG G); Internet homepage: http://www.cabi.org; E-mail: cabi@cabi.org

AGRIS

The AGRIS (International Information System for Agricultural Sciences and Technology) database is managed by the Library and Documentation Systems Division of FAO, Rome. The database is compiled from information provided by 158 national and 28 regional and international input centres around the world and contains nearly 3 million bibliographic records prepared since 1975. Subject areas covered include all aspects of agriculture, fisheries, human nutrition and management of natural resources and environment.

In addition to scientific literature, the database contains material which cannot easily be found in other databases, compiled from less widely known publications of local or regional relevance. The database can be searched using keywords in several languages with the aid of a multilingual vocabulary. Current rate of input of new records is over 150,000 per year. The database is made available to users through online vendors and CD-ROM suppliers such as DIALOG, DIMDI, ESA-IRS, FAXON, MICROINFO and SILVER PLATTER.

Contact: the nearest national AGRIS centre or WAICENT/FAOINFO, Dissemination Management Branch,1 Via delle Terme di Caracalla, 00100 Rome, Italy. Telephone: (396) 5705 4993; Fax: (396) 5705 4049; Telex: 625852 FAO I; Internet homepage: http://www.fao.org/library/default.htm; E-mail: FAO-Agris-Caris@fao.org

AGRICOLA

Bibliographic database compiled and maintained by the US National Agricultural Library, Beltsville, Maryland. The database contains over 3 million records of post-1970 publications covering all aspects of agriculture and provides particularly extensive coverage of US literature not covered by other agricultural databases (e.g. reports from agricultural experiment stations containing material not published elsewhere). It is made available to users through online and CD-ROM vendors DIALOG, DIMDI, FAXON, MICROINFO, SILVER PLATTER and others.

Contact:: National Agricultural Library, 10301 Baltimore Boulevard, Beltsville, MD 20705-2351, USA. Internet URL:
http://www.nalusda.gov/general_info/agricola/agricola.html

PASCAL

Compiled by the Institut de l'Information Scientifique et Technique (INIST) of the French Centre National de la Recherche Scientifique, PASCAL is one of the world's largest multidisciplinary bibliographic information databases covering literature published in all areas science and technology, including biology and medicine. This French/English bilingual database contains over 12 million records relating to papers published in over 25,000 serials, 56,000 reports, 60,000 conference proceedings and 100,000 theses covering the period from 1973 to date. Current rate of growth is over 500,000 records per year. It provides better coverage of French literature than any other database. Search aids include a lexicon containing over 80,000 descriptors and the lexicon is available in 3 languages, viz. French, English and Spanish.

A sister database called FRANCIS, also compiled by INIST, covers literature in social sciences (including ethnology) and economics.

PASCAL can be accessed online, or offline on CD-ROM, using the services of online and CD-ROM vendors such as QUESTEL/ORBIT, ESA-IRS and DIALOG/DATA STAR.

Contact: INIST DIFFUSION, 2 Allée du Parc de Brabois, 54514 Vandoeuvre Cedex, France. Telephone: +33 83 50 46 64; Fax: +33 83 50 46 66; Internet homepage: http://www.inist.fr

BIOSIS PREVIEWS

Probably the world's largest bibliographic information database on biological subjects including medicine, compiled by BIOSIS of Philadelphia, USA. The database contains over 12 million citations and the current rate of addition of new records is 540,000 per year. As with other databases, the source literature includes journals, books, monographs and conference proceedings. In addition to online access, the database is published for offline consultation on CD-ROMs and in printed form in *Biological Abstracts* and other abstract journals. Subscriptions to these are available through online vendors and CD-ROM distributors.

Contact: BIOSIS, 2100 Arch Street, Philadelphia, PA 19103-1399, USA. Telephone: +1 215-587-4847; Fax: +1 215-587-2016. Internet homepage: http://www.biosis.org

CHEMICAL ABSTRACTS

For phytochemical information on medicinal plants and patent-related literature, *Chemical Abstracts* is an indispensable resource. The CHEMICAL ABSTRACTS database compiled by CAS (a division of the American Chemical Society) in Columbus, Ohio, contains some 13 million abstracts of literature and patents in all areas of chemistry and chemical engineering covering the period from 1970 to date. Over 700,000 new records are added per year. The accompanying CA REGISTRY database contains information on over 16 million chemical substances. The database can be searched online or on CD-ROM. Literature published prior to 1970 can be found in the printed journal *Chemical Abstracts*. Search aids include a very detailed list of indexing terms used.

Online access is provided through the STN International online network. Subscriptions are also available through national offices in many countries. e.g. Royal Society of Chemistry in the UK; VCH Verlagsgesellschaft mbH in Germany, Centre National de l'Information Chimique in France, Japan Association for International Chemical Information in Japan, etc.

Contact: Chemical Abstracts Service, 2540 Olentangy River Road, P O Box 3012, Columbus, Ohio 43210, USA.

Telephone: +1 614 447 3600; Fax: +1 614 447 3713; Internet homepage: http://www.cas.org

MEDLINE

A limited amount of information relating to medicinal plants (from mainstream medical literature) can be found in this most widely known database of medicine compiled by the National Library of Medicine, USA.

The database is available to users through a large number of online and CD-ROM vendors including: BLAISE LINK, CD-PLUS, DATA-STAR, DIALOG, DIMDI, EURO-CD DIFFUSION, FAXON, INFOPRO TECHNOLOGIES, LEARNED INFORMATION LTD, MIC KIBIC, OPTECH LTD, QUESTEL/ORBIT, STN, TELESAMPO etc.

Although direct online searches are still fee-based, free search facilities are now provided by a number of organisations through their websites on the Internet. The CD-ROM is also becoming widely available in public libraries around the world.

Contact: The National Library of Medicine, 8600 Rockville Pike, Bethesda, MD 20894. USA. Telephone: 800-272-4787 or 301-496-6308 Internet homepage: http://www.nlm.nih.gov

EMBASE

Literature published in some 3,600 biomedical journals is covered in this bibliographic database of medicine produced by Elsevier, Amsterdam. It contains some 6.5 million records covering the period from 1974 to date. Products derived from the database include CD-ROMs and the printed journal *Excerpta Medica.* Like MEDLINE, coverage of literature on medicinal plants is restricted to that appearing in mainstream biomedical journals.

The database also accessible through various online and CD-ROM vendors including CD PLUS, DATA-STAR, DIALOG, DIMDI, FAXON, INFOPRO TECHNOLOGIES, MICROINFO; SILVER PLATTER and STN.

Contact: Elsevier Science B.V., P O Box 211, 1000 AE Amsterdam, The Netherlands.
Telephone: +31 20 485 3757; Fax: +31 20 485 3432; Internet homepage: http://www.elsevier.nl

Tertiary information databases

Unlike the secondary information databases listed above, tertiary electronic publications containing information on medicinal and related groups of plants vary widely in their design, structure and contents. A number of them, produced for different purposes by various organisations, are listed below in alphabetical order. While some of them can be accessed online, others are only available only on CD-ROM or other offline electronic media.

AHEAD CD-ROM

The Asian Health, Environmental and Allied Databases (AHEAD) CD-ROM series consists of 3 disks containing various databases contributed by the participating organisations based in India, Thailand, Philippines, Malaysia, Singapore and Bangladesh. The project is sponsored by the International Development Research Centre of Canada and co-ordinated by the National Institute of Science Communication (NISCOM), New Delhi (formerly known as PID, Publications and Information Directorate of the Indian Council of Scientific and Industrial Research).

Disk 1 entitled "Environment Asia" contains full-text and bibliographic databases related to water management, recycling of waste water, hygiene education and community participation. Disk 2, named "Wealth Asia", contains the entire *Medicinal and Aromatic Plants* bibliographic database mentioned above and a full-text database of Indian plant, animal and mineral resources, based on the well known "Wealth of India" encyclopaedic book series. Disk 3 is called "Health Asia" and contains a bibliographic database on tropical (mosquito-transmitted) diseases and occupational safety and health, a full-text database on water-borne (diarrhoeal) diseases, and a natural toxins database providing text and pictorial information on poisonous plants and animals.

Contact: The Executive Director, AHEAD, NISCOM, Dr K S Krishnan Marg, New Delhi 110012, India. Telephone: New Delhi 572 8385; Fax: New Delhi 578 7062; Telex: 031-7721; E-mail: pid@sirnetd.ernet.in

APINMAP

The Asian Pacific Information Network on Medicinal and Aromatic Plants (APINMAP) is a UNESCO-sponsored voluntary network of organisations in 14 Asian and Pacific region countries (Australia, People's Republic of China, India, Indonesia, Republic of Korea, Malaysia, Nepal, Pakistan, Papua New Guinea, the Philippines, Sri Lanka, Thailand, Turkey and Vietnam) with a Secretariat based in the Philippines. Its objective is to promote exchange of information relating to medicinal and aromatic plants between its member organisations. Databases and other resources held by each organisation are shared with others. APINMAP resources include an Integrated APINMAP database containing bibliographic and factual information on medicinal plants, lists of research projects, institutions and personnel. Other databases shared include the AHEAD CD-ROM series mentioned above, the Health Research and Development Information Network (**HERDIN**) database from the Philippines and the **FLOTURK** database (see below) from Turkey.

Contact: Secretary General, APINMAP, Philippine Council for Health Research and Development, Department of Science and Technology, Bicutan, Tagig, Metro Manila, Philippines. Telephone: Manila 837-29-42. Internet homepage: http://www.pchrd.dost.gov.ph/apinmap/

BACIS

Boelens Aroma Chemical Information Service (BACIS) offers a set of five databases (which can be installed on a desktop PC) mainly aimed at users in the perfumery and flavouring industries. These contain information on volatile compounds in foods, analytical chemical data compiled from published literature on essential oils and other natural compounds, and trade-related data.

Contact: BACIS, Groen van Prinstererlaan 21, 1272 GB Huizen, The Netherlands. Telephone and Fax: +31 2152 53558

BIOLOGICALLY ACTIVE PHYTOCHEMICALS AND THEIR ACTIVITIES; and

PHYTOCHEMICAL CONSTITUENTS OF GRAS HERBS AND OTHER ECONOMIC PLANTS

A set of two databases compiled by Dr James Duke of ARS/USDA. The first of these contains information on some 3000 biologically active (medicinal, antimicrobial, pesticidal and allelopathic) phytochemicals, their reported activities and inhibitory concentrations or doses. The second database lists the chemical constituents of approximately 1000 plant species. These include most of the GRAS (generally recognised as safe) plants, many medicinally important foods (GRAF, generally recognised as foods) and about 500 strictly medicinal (GRAP, generally recognised as poisonous or medicinal) plants. Quantitative information is included where available. A rather complicated set of codes is used to indicate plant parts and reference sources.

These databases are published in book form with accompanying diskettes, by CRC Press, Inc. Information contained in these databases can be searched online on the **Phytochemical Database** (which also has input from other interconnected databases) on the Internet at the following URL:
http://probe.nalusda.gov:8300/cgi-bin/query?dbname=phytochemdb

Contact: CRC Press Inc., 2000 Corporate Blvd., N.W., Boca Raton, FL 33431, USA.

BRAZILIAN MEDICINAL PLANTS DATABASE

This is a database being developed by the Medicinal Plants Laboratory of the Escola Superior de Agricultura "Luiz de Queiroz", Sao Paulo University, and CIAGRI, the computing centre of the university.

It currently contains the common name in Portuguese, Lain name and synonyms, family, biological activity, and therapeutic uses of over a thousand species.

Contact: ESA "Luiz de Queiroz", Piracicaba, Sao Paulo, Brazil. Internet URL: http://www.ciagri.usp.br/planmedi/planger.htm

CHINA ACADEMY OF TRADITIONAL CHINESE MEDICINE DATABASES

The Institute of Information of the China Academy of Traditional Chinese Medicine has put together several bibliographic and factual information databases. The largest among these is the **Traditional Chinese Medical Literature Analysis and Retrieval System** (TCMLARS), which contains about 200,000 bibliographic records of literature on traditional Chinese medicine, Chinese herbal medicine, integrated traditional Chinese medicine and Western medicine, published in over 500 Chinese and foreign biomedical journals since 1984. TCMLARS consists of its three constituent databases, the largest among these being the **Traditional Chinese Medical Literature** (TCM) database. The other two are the **Acupuncture Literature Analysis and Retrieval System** (ACULARS), and the **Chinese Materia Medica** (CMM) database which contains chemical, pharmacological and horticultural information on medicinal plants. TCMLARS has both English and Chinese versions.

Other databases which are exclusively in Chinese language include a **Traditional Chinese Medical Research Achievement** database, a **TCM News** Database, a **Traditional Chinese Patent Drug and Health Products** database (which contains about 2000 entries relating to the production and marketing of traditional Chinese patent drugs and health products), an **Aids Information** database and an **Overseas TCM Academic Organisations and Scholars** database.

All the above databases can be searched at the institute. A fee-based search service is provided.

Contact: Retrieval Section, Institute of Information on Traditional Chinese Medicine, China Academy of Traditional Chinese Medicine, 18 Beixincang, Dongzhimen Nei, Beijing, 100700, P. R. China. Telephone: (10) 403 2167; Fax: (10) 403 2167; E-mail: wulc@sun.ihep.ac.cn

CHINESE UNIVERSITY OF HONG KONG DATABASES

The Chinese Medicinal Material Research Centre (CMMRC) of the Chinese University of Hong Kong has compiled a database of TCM which contains botanical, chemical, pharmacological and clinical information selected from Chinese medical treatises and translated into English. This database is updated by abstracting papers form over 180 medical and other scientific journals in Chinese.

CMMRC is also developing a database on the safety of Chinese foods and medicines. The first product is CHIMERA, a bibliographic database on reported cases of adverse reactions to Chinese foods and medicines. Colour images of the suspected materials are also included in this database.

Contact: Chinese Medicinal Material Research Centre, The Chinese University of Hong Kong, Hong Kong. E-mail: cmmrc@cuhk.edu.hk

DICTIONARY OF NATURAL PRODUCTS

DNP on CD-ROM published by Chapman and Hall contains chemical, physical, bibliographic and structural data on over 113,000 natural products, organised into over 36,000 entries. Pharmacologically active compounds, food ingredients and many compounds of biochemical significance are well covered. Categories of natural products covered include amino acids, peptides and proteins, antibiotics, nucleosides, alkaloids, terpenoids, flavonoids, lignans, lichen acids, polyacetylenes, tannins and coumarins. In addition to text-based searches using keywords, it offers the possibility of searching by drawing structures or parts of structures of the compounds concerned.

Contact: Chapman and Hall, 2-6 Boundary Row, London SE1 8HN, UK. Telephone: +44 171 865 0066; Fax: +44 171 522 9621. Internet homepage: http://www.thomson.com:8866/chaphall/default.html

DIRECTORY OF SPECIALISTS IN HERBS, SPICES AND MEDICINAL PLANTS

This is a database containing names, addresses, professional expertise and interests, and contact details of specialists in this field, compiled by Professor Lyle Craker, University of Massachusetts, Amherst. It is available in printed form.

Contact: Professor L E Craker, Department of Plant and Soil Sciences, University of Massachusetts, Stockbridge, Amherst, MA 01003, USA. Telephone: +1 413 545 2347; Fax: +1 413 545 1242.

Langer's DROGENANALYSE

published by Deutscher Apotheker Verlag, Stuttgart, Germany, is a plant identification aid database on floppy disk. It contains names, synonyms and illustrations of medicinal and poisonous plants (2,400 entries in total).

Contact: Deutscher Apotheker Verlag, Postfach 10 10 61, 70009 Stuttgart, Germany. Telephone: (0711) 25 82 347 oder 257; Fax: (0711) 25 82 290

ETHMED

is a database currently being compiled at the Yakko Kaiseki Centre (Analytical Research Centre for Ethnomedicines) of the Institute for Wakan-Yaku (Traditional Sino Japanese Medicines) affiliated to the Faculty of Pharmaceutical Sciences of Toyama University, Japan. Data on morphology, anatomy, active principles, biological activity and uses of medicinal plants are being recorded. The project is linked to the cataloguing and indexing of the crude drug samples held at the Museum of Materia Medica of the Institute, which is the largest museum of its kind in the world. The museum holds over 20,000 crude drug samples, more than 75,000 herbarium specimens, and other pharmaceutical preparations covering virtually every system of traditional and folk medicine practised around the world.

Contact: Analytical Research Centre for Ethnomedicines, Research Institute for Wakan-Yaku, Toyama Medical and Pharmaceutical University, 2630 Sugitani, Toyama 930-01, Japan. Fax: 0764-34-5055; Internet homepage: http://www.toyama-mpu.ac.jp

FLAVOUR AND FRAGRANCE MATERIALS

is a chemical entry database published by Allured Publishing Corporation. The database contains 2,500 records with CAS registry numbers, structure, molecular formulae and physical constants for flavour and fragrance materials.

Contact: Allured Publishing Corporation, 362 South Schmale Road, Carol Stream, IL 60188-2787, USA. Telephone: (708) 653 2155; Fax: (708) 653 2192; Internet URL: http://www.barnaby.com/cosmetic.html

FLORIN MEDICINAL PLANTS

FLORIN MEDICINAL PLANTS database is compiled by Professor Boris Golovkin of the Moscow Botanic Gardens. It is one of the several taxonomic and economic botany databases published by Florin, Inc. of Moscow.

FLORIN MEDICINAL PLANTS now contains information on over 5,000 taxa of vascular plants from more than 200 families and is expected to grow to twice its current size in the near future. Taxonomic data, plant parts used, bioactive substances they contain and their therapeutic activity or toxicity are among the interactively searchable fields. Classified lists of diseases and drugs are also included.

Contact: DataX/FLORIN, Inc., Moscow, Russia. Telephone: (095)158-9520; Fax: (095)158-5700: Internet homepage: http://www.florin.ru

FLOTURK

FLOTURK (FLOra of TURKey) is a database compiled and maintained by the Anadolu University Medicinal Plant and Drug Research Centre (TBAM). It contains botanical, phytochemical, chemotaxonomic and pharmacological activity-related data as well as information on production and commercial potential of Turkish flora.

Contact: Anadolu University Medicinal Plant and Drug Research Centre, Eskisehir 26470, Turkey. Telephone: +90 222 335 2952; Fax: +90 222 335 0127; Internet hompage:http://www.anadolu.edu.tr/anadolu/tbam/index.html

GREEN MEDICINE

is a Chinese Herbal Medicine database containing information on 390 biomedical syndromes, 257 basic formulas, 490 individual herbs and 600 variations.

Contact: The Journal of Chinese Medicine, 22 Cromwell Road, Hove, Sussex, England. Fax: +44 1273 748588

HOPKINS TECHNOLOGY CD-ROMs

The series of multimedia CD-ROMs published by Hopkins Technology of Hopkins, Minnesota, include (1) the **HERBALIST** and (2) the **TRADITIONAL CHINESE MEDICINE AND PHARMACOLOGY** databases.

The HERBALIST by David Hoffman is an encyclopaedia of western herbal medicine and gives botanical information on the plants used as well as medical and pharmacological information relating to their use. The *Materia Medica* consists of data sheets on some 170 plant species illustrated with colour pictures and containing the following information: Latin and common names, method of collection, parts used, constituents, pharmacological activity, preparations and dosage.

The TRADITIONAL CHINESE MEDICINE & PHARMACOLOGY CD-ROM describes the basic philosophical elements, and diagnostic and therapeutic principles of TCM. The *Materia Medica* gives information on the use of 322 medicinal herbs with colour illustrations. Commonly used formulas are given with their functions and applications.

Contact: Hopkins Technology, LLC, 421 Hazel Lane, Hopkins, MN 55343-7116, USA. Telephone: (612) 931 9376; Fax: (612) 931 9377. Internet homepage: http://www.hoptechno.com/

ILDIS WORLD DATABASE OF LEGUMES

This database being compiled by the INTERNATIONAL LEGUME DATABASE & INFORMATION SERVICE (ILDIS) is a major source of information on leguminous plants, many of which have medicinal uses. Many institutions around the world participate in this project managed by Dr Frank Bisby of the Biology Department, University of Southampton. The database consists of an exhaustive checklist of species of the Fabaceae with names and synonyms, geographic distribution, life-form and conservation data, known economic uses and key literature citations. Combining taxonomic data from this database with phytochemical data from the Chapman & Hall *Dictionary of Organic Compounds* has led to the publication of the book *Phytochemical Dictionary of the Leguminosae.* Further expansion of this database by including root nodulation data and interlinking it with ethnobotanical and molecular biological datasets has been planned.

Subscriptions for online searches are available through BIDS at Bath University, UK. The online version is called **LegumeLine**.

Contact: Bioinformatics Laboratory, Biology Department, University of Southampton, Southampton SO9 3TU, UK. Internet homepage: http://molbiol.soton.ac.uk/~biology/ildis/index.html

INMEDPLAN

INMEDPLAN (Indian Medicinal Plants National Network of distributed databases) is an initiative of a network of several Indian organisations with expertise on different aspects of medicinal plants to build a multidisciplinary (botanical, horticultural, pharmacological and other) information pool by sharing their resources. The network secretariat is at FRLHT, Bangalore.

Contact: Foundation for Revitalisation of Local Health Traditions, 50 MSH Layout, Anandnagar, Bangalore 560 024, India. Telephone: +91 80 333 6909; Fax: +91 80 333 4167; Internet homepage: http://ece.iisc.ernet.in/ernet-members/frlht.html

MAPI

MAPI (Major Aromatic Plants of India) is a database compiled by the Central Institute of Medicinal and Aromatic Plants, Lucknow. It contains very detailed botanical, agronomic, phytochemical and bibliographic information on 45 major aromatic plants of India. The database has a very elaborate structure with a total of 86 unique data entry fields for each record.

Contact: Central Institute of Medicinal and Aromatic Plants, P B No. 1, RSM Nagar, Lucknow 226016, India.

Telephone: +91 522 71170; Fax: +91 522 73654; Internet homepage: http://www.sunsite.sut.ac.jp/asia/india/jitnet/india/csir/cimap.html

MEDICINAL PLANTS OF MALTA

An electronic inventory of 300 medicinal and aromatic plants of Malta, compiled by the University of Malta, containing text and images.

Contact: Royal University of Malta, Msida, Malta.

MEDICINAL PLANTS OF PAPUA NEW GUINEA

developed by the Wau Ecology Institute Herbarium, this database contains botanical, phytochemical and ethnopharmacological information on plants native to PNG.

Contact: Wau Ecology Institute, P O Box 77, Wau, Papua New Guinea.

NAPRALERT, MEDFLOR and DEREP

These are three inter-related databases developed by the Department of Medicinal Chemistry and Pharmacognosy of the College of Pharmacy, University of Illinois at Chicago, USA.

The **NAPRALERT** (NAtural PRoducts ALERT) database contains bibliographic and factual data on natural products of plant, microbial and animal origin. It is compiled from ethnomedical source literature scanned from some 125,000 journal articles, books, abstracts and patents covering the period from 1975 to date. Some information derived from older literature dating back to 1650 is also included. The database has an elaborate field structure and provides extensive information on the chemistry, pharmacology, biological activity, taxonomic and geographical distribution and ethno-medical uses of some 110,000 natural products and 120,000 organisms. Information from approximately 600 new articles scanned are added every month.

MEDFLOR (MEDicinal FLORa) is an ethnobiological database being developed in collaboration with the Organization of American States. It aims to compile botanical information and ethnomedical uses of plants from literature scanned locally at data entry sites located in Costa Rica, Panama, Trinidad and Tobago, Hungary and India.
DEREP (DEREPlication) is a recently initiated database exclusively containing data on the physical constants of natural products.

Online search subscriptions to NAPRALERT are available through STN International and other online vendors. A CD-ROM version of NAPRALERT has been announced for 1997 by Chapman and Hall. Access to MEDFLOR and DEREP is restricted to collaborating organisations.

Contact: Program for Collaborative Research in the Pharmaceutical Sciences, College of Pharmacy, University of Illinois at Chicago, Chicago, Illinois 60680
Telephone: +1 312-996-5381; Fax: +1 312-996-7107. Internet homepage: http://pcog8.pmmp.uic.edu/mcp/MCP.html

NATTS

NATTS is the Natural Products database developed by the Central Drug Research Institute, Lucknow. It contains factual information on medicinal plants. Detailed data on botanical characters, collection site details, pharmacological screening results, chemical structures of active constituents, uses in folk medicine and in established traditional medicine, information from traditional health systems' literature and from modern scientific literature are recorded in the six sub-files constituting the database.

Contact: Documentation and Library Services Division, Central Drug Research Institute, Chattar Manzil Place, Lucknow 226 001, India. Telephone: Lucknow 234219; Telegram: CENDRUG, LUCKNOW; Telex: 0535-286/0535-344 CDRI IN; Email: cdrilk@sirnetd.ernet.in

PLANTES MEDICINALES

This multimedia CD-ROM database developed as an educational tool by Professor Michel Paris of the Department of Pharmacognosy, Faculty of Pharmacy, Châtenay-Malabry, France is sponsored by the French Ministry of Education and published by Algo Vision, Paris. It contains botanical and phytotherapeutic information on some 175 species and is well illustrated with over 500 high quality colour photographs. Descriptions of pathological conditions are accompanied by monographs on the main species used in the treatment and additional lists of other relevant plants. The French version is expected to become available by June 1997. An English version is also being planned.

Contact: Société ALGO VISION, 27 rue du Château d'eau, 75010 Paris, France. Telephone: +33 1 44 84 03 03; Fax: +33 1 44 84 06 13. E-mail: algovisi@pratique.fr

POISONOUS PLANTS IN BRITAIN AND IRELAND

This is a CD-ROM database developed jointly by the Poisons Unit of Guy's & St Thomas' Hospital Trust, London and the Royal Botanic Gardens, Kew. It is an interactive database designed for identifying common poisonous plants using easily recognisable morphological features such as size, shape and colour of different plant parts for characterising the species concerned. The database contains textual and pictorial information on over 200 plant groups covering approximately 2,000 species and cultivars.

Two versions have been published, a medical version for the benefit of medical professionals dealing with suspected plant poisoning cases, especially in hospital Accidents & Emergency Departments for identifying plants ingested accidentally by children, and a more popular version aimed at the general public.

Contact: The Stationery Office, Electronic Publishing Sales, 51 Nine Elms Lane, London SW8 5DR, UK. Telephone: +44 171 873 8236; Fax: +44 171 873 8203. URL: http://194.128.65.2/publicat/titles/plants/plants.htm

PROSEA

PROSEA (PLANT RESOURCES OF SOUTH-EAST ASIA) is a foundation with an international charter and consists of a network of participating organisations based in Indonesia, Malaysia, Papua New Guinea, Philippines, Thailand, Vietnam and the Netherlands. The network has a secretariat is at Bogor, Indonesia, and a publishing office at Wageningen, Netherlands.

The main objective of PROSEA is to collect and disseminate information on the plant resources of South-East Asia for education, extension, research and industry. Its main activities therefore involve developing electronic databases and publishing books, CD-ROMs, bibliographies etc.

The PROSEA database already contains a wealth of information on some 6,000 useful plants of South-East Asia. A series of scholarly handbooks, CD-ROMs and bibliographies on several commodity groups, and other products derived from the database have already been published. Future publications will include volumes on spices and condiments, medicinal and poisonous plants, essential oil plants, stimulants, and plants producing exudates among others.

Contact: PROSEA Network Office, c/o Research and Development Centre for Biology (RDCB-LIPI), Jalan Ir. H. Juanda 22, P.O.Box 234, Bogor 16122, Indonesia . Telehone: +62 251 322859; Fax: +62 251 370934

or

PROSEA Publication Office, Wageningen Agricultural University (WAU), Haarweg 333, P.O.Box 341, 6700 AH Wageningen, The Netherlands. Telephone: +31 317 484587; Telex: 45917 BURLU; Fax: +31 317 482206; Internet homepage: http://www.bib.wau.nl/prosea/home.html

SEPASAL

The SEPASAL (SURVEY OF ECONOMIC PLANTS FOR ARID AND SEMI-ARID LANDS) database developed by the Centre for Economic Botany, Royal Botanic Gardens, Kew, is a major source of information on the flora of arid and semi-arid regions and a valuable resource for people involved in biodiversity conservation, germplasm collection and storage, and environmental management.

It contains information gathered from various sources on some 6,000 useful dryland species. The data include detailed botanical descriptions, geographic distribution, conservation status, soil and climatic preferences, and uses of different plant parts (following an international standard classification). The range of information and the amount of data vary between species.

Contact: Centre for Economic Botany, Royal Botanic Gardens, Kew, Richmond, Surrey TW9 3AE, UK. Telephone: +44 181 332 5719; Fax: +44 181 332 5278; Internet homepage: http://www. rbgkew.org.uk/ceb/ceb.html

TRADIMED

TRADIMED is a TCM database developed by the Natural Products Research Institute of the Seoul National University. The database contains pharmacological data (efficacy, dosages, adverse effects) for traditional Korean and Chinese drugs, chemical data (composition and structural formulae) for natural products from botanical, microbial and marine organisms, and colour images of medicinal plants. An English version of the database is available on CD-ROM.

Contact: Natural Products Research Institute, Seoul National University, 28 Yeongun-Dong, Jongro-Ku, Seoul 110-460, Republic of Korea. Telephone: +82 2 740 8901; Fax: +82 2 742 9951;URL: http://yes.snu.ac.kr/TradiMedENG.htm

Concluding remarks

With the exception of agronomic literature on a limited number of herbs, spices and condiments, the bulk of the literature on medicinal plants currently available in electronic form appears to be inspired by the objective of identifying new plants containing bioactive compounds or isolating and characterising the active principles from plants already used in herbal therapy in some part of the world. Only an insignificant fraction of the digital information available on major databases relates to the therapeutic use of these plants in the traditional system of medicine from which they were identified in the first place. For example, a substantial amount of phytochemical literature to be found in a number of databases on plants used in traditional Chinese, Ayurvedic, or western herbal medicine, is generated from screening programmes and other studies aimed at isolating bioactive molecules. Yet, the same databases contain virtually no information on the conditions under which these plants are already being used effectively in the traditional system of medicine concerned.

As mentioned above, a certain amount of information on traditional Chinese medicine is now becoming available in electronic form through the databases from China, Hong Kong and Korea. Literature on other established systems of traditional and folk medicine from around the world is yet to make its appearance on electronic media.

It is encouraging to note that the Internet is becoming increasingly popular among herbalists and practitioners of herbal medicine in the West. The volume of information available on Western herbal medicine on the Internet is therefore rapidly increasing. However, the impact of the widening gap in access to information technology between different parts of the world on the way in which information originating from traditional knowledge held by indigenous peoples and cultures around the world is disseminated and used remains to be seen.

Reference

Bhat, K. K. S. 1995. Literature published during the past two decades on medicinal, aromatic and other related groups of plants. *Acta Horticulturae* 390: 11-17.

Part two: Articles on Regional Aspects of Medicinal Plants Use

Biodiversity - People Interface in Nepal

Nirmal K. Bhattarai
Scientific Officer, National Herbarium
G.P.O. Box 938, Kathmandu, Nepal
Tel. 977-1-413396 Fax: 977-1-225603
Email: CCSL@casnov.attmail.com

Abstract

The flora of Nepal consist of some 7,000 species of vascular plants of which 252 are endemic. There are more than 75 vegetation types spread across an area of 147,181 square kilometres. About 14 per cent of the area of the country has been brought under protection. More than 700 species of medicinal plants grow wild in the country, majority of which are used in folk herbal remedies. Every year, over fifteen thousand tons of medicinal herbs representing some 100 species are harvested from the wild for commercial and industrial purposes.

Useful wild plants of the Nepal Himalaya are of critical importance to hundreds of thousands of rural people as sources of nutrition, health care, raw materials and cash income. The interaction between these people and the wild plant resources has emerged as the most important factor in sustaining the region. In Nepal, quantitative analyses of the effect of extraction on natural plant population are lacking. Indiscriminate collection, not in accordance with any regulatory procedure or recognised management practices, has threatened the survival of some species and reduced the quality of many wild species.

The threat to biodiversity originates from the activities of the rural communities suffering from ignorance, poverty and lack of employment opportunities. Therefore, a key aspect of any campaign for the conservation and sustainable use of biological resources is enhancing community awareness and participation. Sustainable development and biodiversity conservation must be firmly linked if Nepal is to assure the conservation of its natural resources and meet the needs and improve the quality of life of its present population and future generations.

Introduction

Nepal, with a population of about 21 million, extends over a distance of some 800 km along the great Himalayan range in the south-easterly direction from 81° 15' to 88° 10' E. The total area is 147,181 square kilometres and the altitude ranges from 60 to 8,848 m above mean sea level. With the widest altitudinal variation in the world within the narrow width of about 150-200 km, Nepal is endowed with at least 75 vegetation types and a rich flora, estimated at about 7,000 species of higher plants.

As Nepal occupies the central part of the great Himalayan range, its flora lie in a transition zone between the flora of west Himalaya containing many west Himalayan elements, and that of east Himalaya, with many Sino-Japanese elements. It also harbours plants representative of the Tibetan plateau in its many northern frontiers, especially in the trans-Himalayan regions. Numerous plants representative of the Indo-Gangetic plains are also found in its tropical regions. Plant diversity in Nepal can also be illustrated from the fact that over 1000 species of Himalayan plants have originally been discovered and described from the Nepalese flora. (Bajracharya *et al.*, 1988). Nepal's floral diversity contains some 370 endemic plant species (Joshi and Joshi, 1991) of which 252 are higher plants (Bajracharya *et al.*, 1988).

Nepal's commitments to biodiversity conservation for sustainable development

Nepal was an active participant at the UN Conference on Human Environment held in Stockholm in 1972. It is also involved with the United Nations Environmental Program (UNEP) as an elected member of its Governing Council since 1984. Nepal, as one of the signatories of the Rio Declaration, is firmly committed to the protection of the environment by an effective national action plan with particular concern and interest on matters relating to the conservation of biological diversity and improvement of the living conditions of the poor. Besides, Nepal has entered into a number of obligations and co-operative agreements related to conservation. It is a signatory to the Convention concerning the Protection of the World Cultural and Natural Heritage (World Heritage Convention) which it accepted on 20 June 1978. Two natural sites, Sagarmatha (Mt. Everest) and Royal Chitwan National Park, have since been inscribed on the World Heritage List. Fourteen protected areas including the national parks and other wildlife reserves have so far been established, covering about 14 per cent of land area of the country.

The new Constitution of the Kingdom of Nepal-1991 formally recognises the need to preserve the environment and to use natural resources wisely. At present, six non-timber forest products (NTFPs) which are recognised as threatened with over-exploitation, are banned from export in unprocessed form: Jatamansi (*Nardostachys grandiflora* DC.), Sugandhawal (*Valeriana jatamansi* Jones), Sugandhakokila (*Cinnamomum glaucescens* (Nees) Drury), Sarpagandha (*Rauvolfia serpentina* Benth. ex Kurz), Jhyau (consisting of several species of Lichens: *Parmelia*, *Ramalina*, *Usnea*, etc.) and the mineral Silajit (a natural form of asphalt). Concerning two other species, *viz.* Panchaunle (*Dactylorhiza hatagirea* (D.Don) Soo) and Yarsagumba (the fungus *Cordyceps sinensis* (Berk.) Sacc.), even their collection is banned.

Sources of threat to biodiversity conservation

The following human activities can be enumerated as the principal threats to conservation of biodiversity in the country:

Deforestation

Tropical hardwood has dominated the trade based on natural resources in Nepal for more than a century. However, this trend has very recently declined because of the depletion of timber reserves from the natural forest through logging and conversion of forest land to other uses. Wood is the principal source of fuel in the country. Over 87 per cent of the nation's energy requirement is met by forest products and each person consumes one cubic meter of wood per year for this purpose (Upreti, 1985).

Population pressure and the so-called developmental activities are causing a rapid depletion of forests in every part of the country. As a result, countless plant species are facing considerable danger of extinction. A significant lowering of the upper timber line has resulted from human activities which include conversion of forest to arable land, commercial timber cutting, excessive gathering of timber for domestic use, construction of roads, dams, canals, high-tension electricity lines, etc. These developments occurred largely during the last fifty years and reached their peak very recently.

Forest fires

Occasionally, forests are intentionally set to fire to kill trees to obtain fuel wood and construction materials, and also to extend the area of the adjoining agricultural lands. Forest fires, especially those in the high-altitude pine (*Pinus wallichiana* A.B. Jacks.) forests are set to enhance the growth and yield of the high-priced morel mushrooms (*Morchella conica* L., *M. esculenta* L., etc.). The pastures are regularly subjected to fire to produce tender grasses. Consequently, many valuable herbs flourishing in those habitats are heavily affected. The fire also destroys the alpine butterfly belonging to the genus *Leptropteris* whose larvae are the host for the highly reputed and endangered medicinal fungus *Cordyceps sinensis* (Berk.) Sacc., ultimately threatening the existence of even the fungus. Mostly the fires are beyond control, and result in severe losses destroying the herbs, roots and rhizomes at ground level and even the clumps. Lower branches of tall trees are also seriously affected by the fire. Organic matter in the upper layer of the soil is usually destroyed resulting in the disappearance of many valuable biological species from the area.

Shifting cultivation

The shifting cultivation, called 'khorea phandne', is another form of destruction of habitat. A patch of the climax forest is cleared, burnt and used for farming for some years after which it is abandoned and the farmers shift to another forest area, clearing another patch of the climax vegetation. This practice results in the destruction of a large number of biological species and the abandoned land is mostly succeeded by a fewer number of sporadic species that are quite different from the original vegetal cover.

Overgrazing

The shortage of fodder and other feeding materials has resulted in overgrazing in the pastures and overlopping of fodder trees in the forests. Fodder for the estimated 15 million cattle in the country, which includes important non-timber forest products used by the villagers, is estimated at 5.6 million tons of fodder per year (Upreti, 1985). About three-quarters of the fodder comes from the forest and grassland, thus posing pressing threat to the country's biodiversity (Sigdyal, 1984).

Overexploitation

In Nepal, there are traditional extraction systems in which very little processing of the products occurs in the area in which they are found. The general pattern is to gather, dry, pack and transport out of the region of origin. A major proportion of the non-wood forest products, especially the medicinal and aromatic herbs collected from the wild, is meant for export. Hence, the quantities of different forest products collected are mostly determined by the demand from abroad. At the same time, the local collectors, mostly belonging to the poorer classes of the community, are being attracted by the market prices for some items that have gone through the roof. As a consequence, raw materials are overharvested by the removal, for example, of immature plants, roots, tubers and rhizomes, or by overpruning. As an outside interest dictates the price and quantity of raw materials extracted, a major part of local ecosystem has suffered irreversible harm.

Medicinal plants in trade and industry

The list of Nepalese medicinal plants contains well over 700 species comprising about 10% of the known vascular plant species of the country (Malla and Shakya, 1984). Every year, thousands of tons of medicinal herbs are collected from the forests and pastures, and traded to foreign countries. The trade in medicinal herbs is an important source of revenue for the government and a major source of income for the rural people. About 100 species of medicinal herbs are currently exploited for commercial and industrial purposes (Malla *et al.*, 1995).

A study of the available records revealed that 3,448 tons of herbs were collected for commercial and industrial purposes during the fiscal year 1989/90, followed by 6,217 tons in 1990/91; 3,372 tons in 1991/92; 5,679 tons in 1992/93; and 11,694 tons in 1993/94. Over 90 per cent of the total export is to India with whom trade links have prevailed since times immemorial.

The uncontrolled commercial extraction has significantly eroded the country's medicinal plant resources, and particular species have gradually become more difficult to find in a given locality where they once flourished. Thus the availability of the high-altitude herbs supplying underground parts, e.g. *Aconitum ferox* Wall., *A. heterophyllum* Wall. ex Royle, *A. spicatum* Stapf., *Dactylorhiza hatagirea* (D.Don) Soo, *Daiswa polyphylla* (Sm.) Rafu. var. *wallichii* Hara, *Fritillaria cirrhosa* D.Don, *Nardostachys grandiflora* DC., *Panax pseudoginseng* Wall., *Picrorhiza scrophulariiflora* Pennell, *Podophyllum hexandrum* Royle, *Rheum australe* D.Don, which were once abundant, has declined drastically in recent years. The supplies of middle- and low-altitude herbs like *Asparagus racemosus* Willd., *Dioscorea deltoidea* Wall. ex Griseb., *Rubia manjith* Roxb. *Valeriana jatamansi* Jones, and many epiphytic orchids, notably *Dendrobium densiflorum* Lindl., *D. longicornu* Lindl., and *D. macraei* Lindl., have reduced considerably. Tropical and sub-tropical herbs like *Alstonia scholaris* (L.) R.Br. and *Rauvolfia serpentina* Benth. ex Kurz have already reached near extinction levels in most areas of the country.

In addition to direct export of herbs, many entrepreneurs are taking an interest in processing for industrial uses such as the production of essential oils and ayurvedic medicines involving thousands of tons of crude herbs collected locally. Collection and trade of medicinal herbs and other non-wood forest products provide up to 50 percent of a family's income in certain areas of the country.

Wild plant resources in the livelihood of the rural people

Apart from commercial and industrial uses, the majority of the lay population use wild plants in a variety of ways, the additional uses being for food, folk medicine, fodder, fuel, and a variety of domestic articles. They are also used as sources of dyes, tannins, fibres, gums and resins, for producing agricultural and hunting tools and weapons, and in witchcraft and magic. Some species are also used in worships and religious rituals.

Considering the specific case of health services, in Nepal, like in most other developing countries, due to the shortage of trained manpower and facilities, modern health services have not been provided to the greater part of the rural areas where the majority of the population lives. This sector of the population is therefore largely dependent on the indigenous medicines, especially the folk herbal medicines which have been used and appreciated since prehistoric times. About 85 percent of the rural Nepalese population are said to use these remedies (Dani, 1986). Wild medicinal plants, therefore, play an invaluable role in the health services available to the rural Nepalese population. The interaction between these people and the wild plant resources has, therefore, emerged as a critical factor in sustaining the region. As 14% of the land including most suitable habitats for different species of medicinal plants has been protected, the pressure on other forests and pastures have increased beyond the carrying capacities of the ecosystem in most parts of the country.

Reasons for the excessive extraction of wild plant resources

The improper and excessive exploitation of biological resources leading to habitat destruction and placing threat on biodiversity is largely due to illiteracy, poverty and the shortage of off-farm employment opportunities for the rural population.

Non-timber forest products, especially medicinal and aromatic plants, are regarded as a free commodity to be collected from nature. Consequently, the raw materials are mostly being overharvested. Illiteracy and poverty have forced the rural Nepalese people to continue activities which help them survive in the present but which will cause more severe problems in the future.

Discussion

People living in rural areas constitute more than three quarters of our population of about 21 million, the majority of whom are dependent, partially or wholly, upon the natural plant resources for their livelihood. The wild plant wealth of the Nepal Himalaya has a rich resource base which potentially can contribute to biological, environmental and economic sustainability as well as to development, provided that recognised management practices and adequate regulatory procedures are brought into action.

As a result of population growth, habitat destruction and increasing commercial demand for raw materials, pressure upon the existing forest and pastures is ever increasing. Consequently, the quantity of wild medicinal plants extracted throughout the country is significant both in terms of volume and economic value. Hence, the great diversity of wild plant resources, which provides the raw materials for Nepal's major industries and serves as the source of livelihood to the rural people, is in deep trouble.

Many plant species which are among commodities traded internationally, have not even been the subject of proper scientific identification. Some prominent examples are 'Amphi', 'Bompo', 'Dhawa', 'Halik', 'Hiunkhamar', 'Kaldana', 'Kawala', 'Mujoseda', 'Rishimarka', 'Sankhadurlabha', 'Sugandhapatta', 'Tairi', and 'Tigedi'. Scientific identification of plants collected and traded is a prerequisite for evaluating their current and potential uses, for initiating conservation measures and for introducing development and management practices effectively.

More than 90 per cent of the non-wood forest products collected for commercial purposes finds its way to India. The species exported include some which are considered threatened or even endangered in India, notably *Aconitum ferox* Wall. ex Seringe, *Allium stracheyi* Baker, *Begonia rubella* Buch.-Ham. ex D. Don, *Cypripedium cordigerum* D. Don, *Dioscorea deltoidea* Wall. ex Griseb., *Nardostachys grandiflora* DC., *Panax pseudo-ginseng* Wall. and *Picrorhiza scrophulariiflora* Pennell among others. Further, most medicinal and aromatic herbs exported to India are re-exported to other countries either in the crude form or after primary processing, in addition to being used in the Indian pharmaceutical industries.

The existing record keeping system in many District Forest Offices and Customs offices is far from satisfactory. It is likely that the quantities of plant material actually collected and exported are significantly greater than the quantities recorded (Malla *et al.*, 1993). Overharvesting is not restricted to products that are collected for commercial markets. Browder (1992) cites many examples from South America of NTFPs used primarily by local communities that are also being depleted by unsustainable extraction, and Nepal is no exception.

The collection of medicinal herbs and other non-timber forest products has generated considerable employment opportunities in remote areas where majority of the people are poor. The common property characteristic of medicinal herbs and other NTFPs also has relevance to the manner in which they are commercially exploited. The collectors most often come from the poorest classes who depend heavily on wild herbs for subsistence. Indiscriminate collection, not in accordance with any regulatory procedure or recognised management practice, has threatened the survival of some species and reduced the quality of many wild species.

Although the exploitation of some plant parts (e.g. fruits, seeds and latex) is less damaging than others (e.g. bark, stems or roots), almost any form of harvesting has an impact on the structure and function of plant populations. There are ways to exploit the non-timber resources produced by plant populations with the minimum of ecological damage. Doing so, however, requires management. Baseline data about the size-class structure and yield characteristics of the population must be collected, regeneration surveys must be conducted, harvest levels must be periodically adjusted, and, in some cases, remedial treatments such as enrichment planting or weeding must be initiated. In Nepal, although there is considerable evidence for overharvesting of medicinal plants, quantitative analyses of the effect of extraction on natural populations are lacking. Without such analyses, it is impossible to assess the effect of harvesting on depletion of resources in natural communities, nor is it possible to design appropriate conservation and management plans.

Recognising that a major proportion of Nepal's biodiversity exists outside of protected areas and that protected areas alone are inadequate to conserve the country's biodiversity, the conservation, development and sustainable use of biological resources outside the protected areas are highly desirable. Regarding protected areas, the objective of Agenda 21 of the Rio Convention (UNCED, 1992) , *viz.* "The first beneficiaries of the conservation and sustainable use of wild plant and animal species should be the rural communities and indigenous people whose traditional knowledge and respect for those resources has preserved them for centuries", is particularly relevant.

At the community level, local people are the true resource managers, with a vested interest in maintaining the natural resources on which they depend. The success of conservation and sustainable use of resources, therefore, largely depends upon the understanding of the people and their acceptance of the concept. As most rural people are ignorant of the needs for environmental conservation, conservation education should be introduced as part of the curriculum in schools and in adult literacy programs. Environmental education needs to focus on the poor and teach practical skills to make people more self-reliant and aware of how to use their local resources sustainably and more profitably.

In Nepal where the overwhelming concern of majority of the population is meeting their immediate needs, it is difficult to conserve and direct resources for the benefit of future generations. The excessive collection of wild plant resources by the rural Nepalese people is therefore not just a case of preference but a situation of having no other option (Bhattarai and Croucher, 1996). The improper and excessive exploitation of medicinal plant resources leading to habitat destruction and threat to biodiversity is, no doubt, the direct outcome of ignorance, poverty and shortage of off-farm employment opportunities. The resource-poor people generally take the view that "If I don't pick what I can today, someone else will get it tomorrow". As a result, even the protected areas like the national parks are facing the problem of indiscriminate collection of plant resources (Yonzon, 1993). These trends and attitudes have led to a cycle of impoverishment in which the local people increasingly loose control over the management of their resources.

Nepal is passing through its eighth five-year plan. The forestry sector has always received increased priority in every plan. In spite of this, the forestry sector has failed to make sufficient progress towards protecting the forests and implementing measures for their sustainable development and management. Even after the vast and uncontrolled deforestation, the mistake of regarding tree plantations as equivalent to natural forest vegetation is unfortunately being repeated. A forest is a community of living beings in which the tree is the most important member. There are trees of different species and of different ages. Bushes, grasses, herbs, insects, birds and wild animals live in this community. They support each other. Such a community cannot grow in monoculture plantations. So the urgent need of the hour is to protect the remaining forests.

The conclusion is a challenge. Our approach to conserve biodiversity for sustainable development should be targeted at different levels, from improving living standards to changing the attitude of the people. If the Himalayan medicinal plants are to continue to serve the needs of the people without being reduced to a dangerously unstable resource base, they have to be considered in the perspective of sound ecological management that also has economic benefits to the local people. Poverty alleviation and biodiversity conservation must be firmly linked if Nepal is to meet the needs and improve the quality of life of its present population and future generations.

Finally, it is worth citing here the opinion expressed by Marco Flores Rodas, the then Assistant Director General of FAO, in the Third World Conference on National Parks: "Until the rural people are ensured adequate food and shelter and a dignified standard of living, all efforts to establish and manage national parks and protected areas will be futile" (Uprety, 1985).

References

Bajracharya, D.M., Joshi, R.M., Rajbhandari, K.R., Shakya, P.R. & Shrestha, T.B. 1988. *Endemism in Nepal flora. In: Proceedings of the National Conference on Science and Technology*. Kathmandu, Nepal; Royal Nepal Academy of Science and Technology. pp. 73-76.

Bhattarai, N.K. & Croucher, J. 1996. Viability of local commercialization of non-timber forest products as a strategy for promoting biodiversity conservation. In: P.K. Jha, G.P.S. Ghimire, S.B. Karmacharya, S.R. Baral & P. Lacoul (Eds). *Environment and Biodiversity : In the Context of South Asia*. Kathmandu, Nepal; Ecological Society. pp.346-353.

Browder, J.O. 1992. Social and economic constraints on the development of market-oriented extractive reserves in Amazon rain forests. In: D.C. Nepstad & S. Schwartzman (Eds). *Non-timber Products from Tropical Forests : Evaluation of a Conservation and Development Strategy. Advances in Economic Botany 9*. Bronx, NY; USA; The New York Botanical Garden. pp. 33-42.

Dani, D.D. 1986. Population and society in Nepal: An overview. In: S.C. Joshi (Ed). *Nepal Himalaya: Geo-ecological Perspective*. Nainital, India; Himalayan Research Group. pp. 163-173.

Joshi, A.R. & Joshi, D.P. 1991. Endemic plants of Nepal Himalaya: Conservation status and future direction. *Mountain Environment and Development* 1: (2) 1-35.

Malla, S.B., Shakya, P.R., Rajbjandari, K. R., Bhattarai, N. K. & Subedi, M.N. 1995. *Minor Forest Products of Nepal : General Status and Trade*. Forest Resource Information System Project Paper No. 4, Forestry Sector Institutional Strengthening Program. Kathmandu, Nepal; Ministry of Forest and Soil Conservation.

Malla, S.B. & Shakya, P.R. 1984. Medicinal plants. In: T.C. Majupuria (Ed). *Nepal - Nature's Paradise*. Bangkok, Thailand; White Lotus Co. Ltd. pp. 261-297.

Sigdyal, K.P. 1984. Save ecological balance. In: T.C. Majupuria (Ed). *Nepal - Nature's Paradise*. Bangkok, Thailand; White Lotus Co. Ltd. pp. 378-382.

UNCED. 1992. *Earth Summit 1992: Relevant Materials*. Kathmandu, Nepal; Coalition Nepal.

Upreti, B.N. 1985. The park-people interface in Nepal: problems and new directions. In: J.A. McNeely, J.W. Thorsell & S.R. Chalise (Eds). *People and Protected Areas in the Hindu Kush Himalaya.* Kathmandu, Nepal; King Mahendra Trust for Nature Conservation and International Centre for Integrated Mountain Development. pp. 19-24.

Yonzon, P. 1993. Raiders of the park. *Himal* 6:(1) 22-23.

Beyond the Biodiversity Convention:
the challenges facing the biocultural heritage of India's medicinal plants

Darshan Shankar and B. Majumdar
Foundation for Revitalisation of Local Health Traditions (FRLHT)
No. 50 MSH Layout, Anandnagar
Bangalore-24, INDIA
Phone : 333 6909, 333 0348 Fax : +91-80-333 4167
E-mail : root@frlht.ernet.in

FRLHT is engaged in one of the most comprehensive efforts being implemented in India to 'conserve' medicinal plants in their natural habitats. Its work is supported through a bilateral aid agreement between the Government of India and DANIDA. FRLHT is concerned not only with the question of conserving the medicinal plant diversity but also its associated cultural diversity. India has one of the richest and oldest, unbroken bio-cultural heritage related to medicinal plants.

Introduction

It cannot be denied that the initiative for the biodiversity convention was a northern initiative, one inspired by two compelling needs: First, a sense of insecurity due to the precarious nature of the planet's ecology (caused, in the first place, almost entirely by the western model of unsustainable development); and second, a desire to have access to the South's abundant biogenetic resources.

The South has reacted to the North's agenda by asking for financial compensations to conserve its tropical forests and has demanded transfer of the North's biotechnology on favourable terms. The North has accepted some of the South's demands after hard bargaining and negotiations are still going on.

Amidst these negotiations on biodiversity conservation and its high-tech utilisation, we in the South seem to have paid insufficient attention to the fact that millions of our people have traditionally been using biodiversity for a wide variety of purposes. Many of these traditional uses have relevance both to our present way of life and to our future well being. As they have a time-tested competence, they are likely to represent the most ecologically sound, safe and sustainable ways of using our bioresources.

India's (and other southern countries') own agenda in biodiversity conservation should not be merely to see on what financial terms access to our biogenetic raw materials should be granted but more importantly to engage creatively in the revitalisation of traditional sciences and technologies, and to use their fruits for the benefit of our own people and to share them on fair terms with the rest of the world.

India's legacy of medicinal plants

The ethos of conserving biodiversity is deeply ingrained in ancient Indian culture. Traditionally, patches of pristine forests were set aside as sacred groves; planting of shade and fruit bearing trees had religious sanction, as also prescriptions to regulate hunting, e.g. ban on killing a pregnant female animal and designating certain parts of the year as closed season. This serious concern for ecology continued to thrive side by side with developments related to economic progress, international trade, and science and technology. In fact the Indian health system which goes back to 1500 BC, and is mainly based on plants and animals, symbolises how deep-rooted was this concern for biodiversity conservation and its sustainable use.

The Indian people know a great deal about medicinal plants. Studies reveal that the largest proportion of the biodiversity in all our ecosystems is used by village communities for human and veterinary health care (See Table 1).

Table 1. An example of uses of biodiversity by "ecosystem people": Some of the medicinal and other plants used by the Mahadev Koli Tribals.*

Purpose	**Number of species**
Medicinal uses	202
Veterinary uses	109
As fish poisons	23
For pest control	51
For water purification	3
As wild edible plants	87
As fodder plants	65
For fuel	30
Hunting purposes	3
Cultural and religious purposes	38

*Source: D. K. Kulkarni Agharkar Institute, Poona.

Over 7,500 species of plants are estimated (AICEP, 1994) to be used by "the ecosystem people" (See Fig. 1) who belong to some 4635 ethnic communities (Anthropological Survey of India, 1994). India probably has the oldest, richest and most diverse, cultural traditions in the use of medicinal plants.

Medicinal plants continue to provide health security to rural people in primary health care (Table 2). According to WHO estimates (Farnsworth and Soejarto, 1991), over 80% of people in developing countries depend on traditional medicines for their primary health needs. In India the coverage of rural population by the modern health system varies between different regions from three to thirty percent (Darshan Shankar, 1992). Thus, for some 4-5 hundred million people, traditional medicine is the only alternative. This is also borne out by the fact that there still exist over one million traditional, village-based carriers of the herbal medicine traditions in the country (LSPSS, 1993).

MEDICINAL PLANTS USED IN FOLK & TRIBAL, AYURVEDA, SIDDHA, UNANI, AMCHI (TIBETAN) AND ALLOPATHIC HEALTH CARE

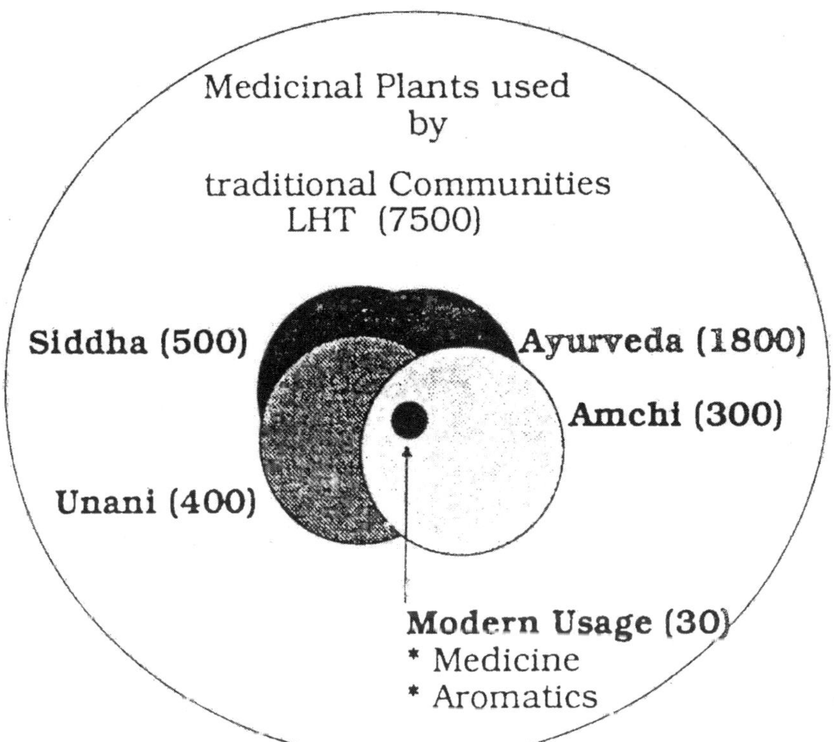

NON INSTITUTION USERS	INSTITUTIONAL USERS
PHYSICIANS	TRADITIONAL PHARMACIES
VETERINARY DOCTORS	PHARMACEUTICALS
FARMERS / COLLECTORS	PERFUMERY INDUSTRY
VILLAGE COMMUNITIES	EXPORTERS
	BOTANICAL GARDENS
	MEDICAL INSTITUTES

Figure 1: Resource base of traditional medicine

Table 2. Richness of folk medicine: Examples of ethno-medicinal plants with ten or more uses reported across ethnic communities in South India.*

Plant species	Reported number of uses
Centella asiatica	33
Pergularia daemia	23
Aristolochia indica	22
Ichnocarpus frutescens	22
Alstonia scholaris	19
Holarrhena antidysenterica	18
Trachyspermum ammi	16
Hygrophila auriculiculata	15
Trianthema portulacastrum	15
Semecarpus anacardium	15
Hemidesmus indicus	15
Catharanthus roseus	14
Apama siliquosa	13
Anacardium occidentale	12
Costus speciosus	12
Justicia gendarussa	11
Pergularia extensa	10

*Source: FRLHT Research Department.

Table 3. List of species banned from export by the Ministry of Commerce (vide notification no. 47 (PN)/92-97 dated 30 March 1994.

Aconitum sp.
Acorus sp.
Angiopteris sp.
Aristolochia sp.
Artemisia sp.
Arundinaria jaunsarensis
Atropa sp.
Balanophora sp.
Berberis aristata (Indian barberry; Rasvat)
Colchicum luteum (Hirantutya)
Commiphora wightii
Coptis sp.
Coscinium fenestratum (Calumba wood)
Costus speciosus (Keu, Kust)
Cyathea gigantea
Cycas beddomei (Beddomes cycad)
Didymocarpus pedicellata
Dioscorea deltoidea
Dolomiaea pedicellata
Drosera sp.
Ephedra sp.
Gentiana kurroo (Kuru, Kutki)
Gloriosa superba
Gnetum sp.
Gynocardia odorata (Chaulmogri)
Hydnocarpus sp.
Hyoscyamus niger (Black henbane)
Iphigenia indica
Meconopsis betonicifolia
Nardostachys sp. (Jatamansi)
Nepenthes khasiana (Pitcher plant)
Osmunda sp.
Paphiopedilium sp. (Ladies' slipper orchid)
Physochlaina praealta (Bajarbang)
Podophyllum hexandrum
Pratia serpumlia
Rauvolfia sp. (Serpgandha)
Renanthera imschootiana (Red vanda)
Rheum emodi (Dolu)
Rhododendron sp.
Saussurea lappa (Kuth)
Strychnos potatorum (Nirmali)
Swertia chirata (Charayatah)
Taxus baccata (Yewu, Birm)
Urginea sp.
Vanda caerulea (Blue vanda)

Table 4. A first red data list of South Indian medicinal plants (based on CAMP report; IUCN version 2.2).

Species	Status*	Species	Status*
Acorus calamus	VU/N &CR/R	*Lamprachaenium microcephalum*	EN
Adenia hondala	VU	*Madhuca diplostemon*	E
Adhatoda beddomei	CR	*Madhuca insignis*	EX
Aegle marmelos	VU	*Michelia champaca*	VU
Aerva wightii	EX	*Moringa concanensis*	VU
Amorphophallus paeonifolius	VU	*Myristica malabarica*	E
Ampelocissus araneosa	VU	*Nervilia aragoana*	EN
Ampelocissus indica	EN	*Nilgirianthus ciliatus*	EN
Andrographis paniculata	LR	*Nothapodytes nimmoniana*	VU
Aristolochia bracteata	LR	*Ochreinauclea missionis*	VU
Aristolochia tagala	VU	*Operculina turpethum*	LR
Artemisia nilagirica	LR	*Oroxylum indicum*	VU
Asparagus rattleri	EX	*Paphiopedilum druryi*	CR
Balanites aegyptiaca	LR	*Phoenix pusilla*	LR
Buchanania lanzan	LR	*Piper barberi*	CR
Cayratia pedata	CR	*Piper longum*	LR
Cleome burmanni	DD	*Piper mullesua*	VU
Commiphora mukul	VU/R	*Piper nigrum*	VU
Coscinium fenestratum	CR	*Plectranthus vetiveroides*	EW
Cycas circinalis	VU& CR/R	*Pterocarpus santalinus*	E
Cyclea fissicalyx	E	*Pseudarthria viscida*	LR
Drosera indica	LR	*Puereria tuberosa*	LR
Drosera peltata	VU	*Rauvolfia serpentina*	E
Elaeagnus conferta	LR	*Saraca asoca*	VU E/R
Embelia ribes	LR	*Schrebera swietenioides*	VU
Garcinia indica	VU	*Symplocos cochinchinensis laurina*	VU
Garcinia morella	VU	*Symplocos racemosa*	LR
Gardenia gummifera	LR	*Syzygium travancoricum*	CR
Glycosmis macrocarpa	LR	*Tinospora sinensis*	VU
Gloriosa superba	LR	*Tragia bicolor*	VU
Hedychium coronarium	LR	*Trichopus zeylanicus*	CR
Heliotropium keralense	EN	*Utleria salicifolia*	CR
Holostemma annulare	VU	*Vateria indica*	LR
Hydnocarpus macrocarpa	VU	*Vateria macrocarpa*	CR
Janakia arayalpathra	CR	*Vernonia anthelmintica*	LR
Kaempferia galanga	CR/R	*Woodfordia fruticosa*	LR
Kingiodendron pinnatum	E		

*CR = Critically endangered; E = Endangered; EX = Extinct; VU = Vulnerable; LR = Low-risk; DD = Data-deficient; EW = Extinct in wild; R = Regional

Source: FRLHT Research Department

Today these biodiversity-dependent rural communities are facing a serious resource threat because of the rapid loss of natural habitats, and the over-exploitation of medicinal plants from the wild (Figs. 2, 3 and 4, and Tables 3 and 4). To meet the demands of the Indian herbal industry which has annual turnover of about US$ 300 million (ADMA, 1996), tons of medicinal plants are being harvested every year from some 165,000 ha of forests (estimates based on extrapolation of regional trade figures by FRLHT Research Department).

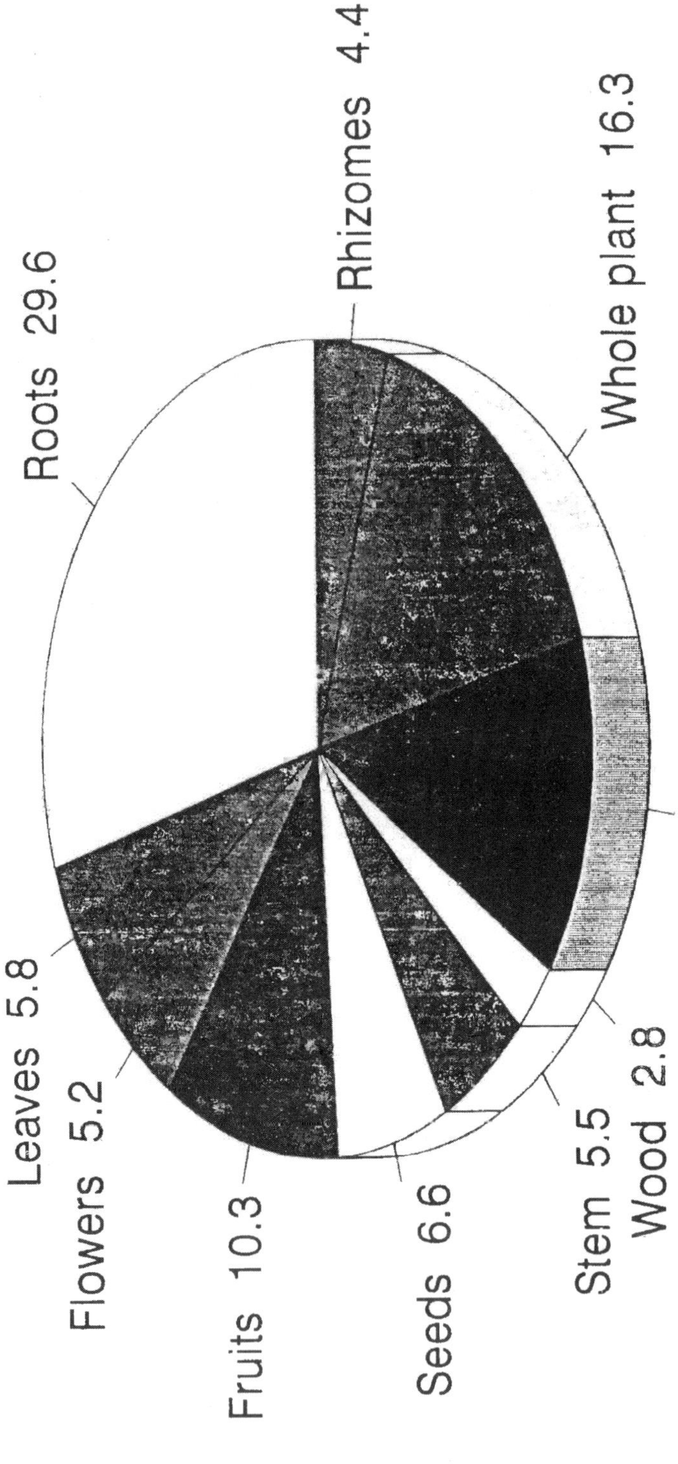

Source : FRLHT Research Department

Figure 2: Destructive collections: distribution of medicinal plants by parts used (72% destructive and 28% non-destructive)

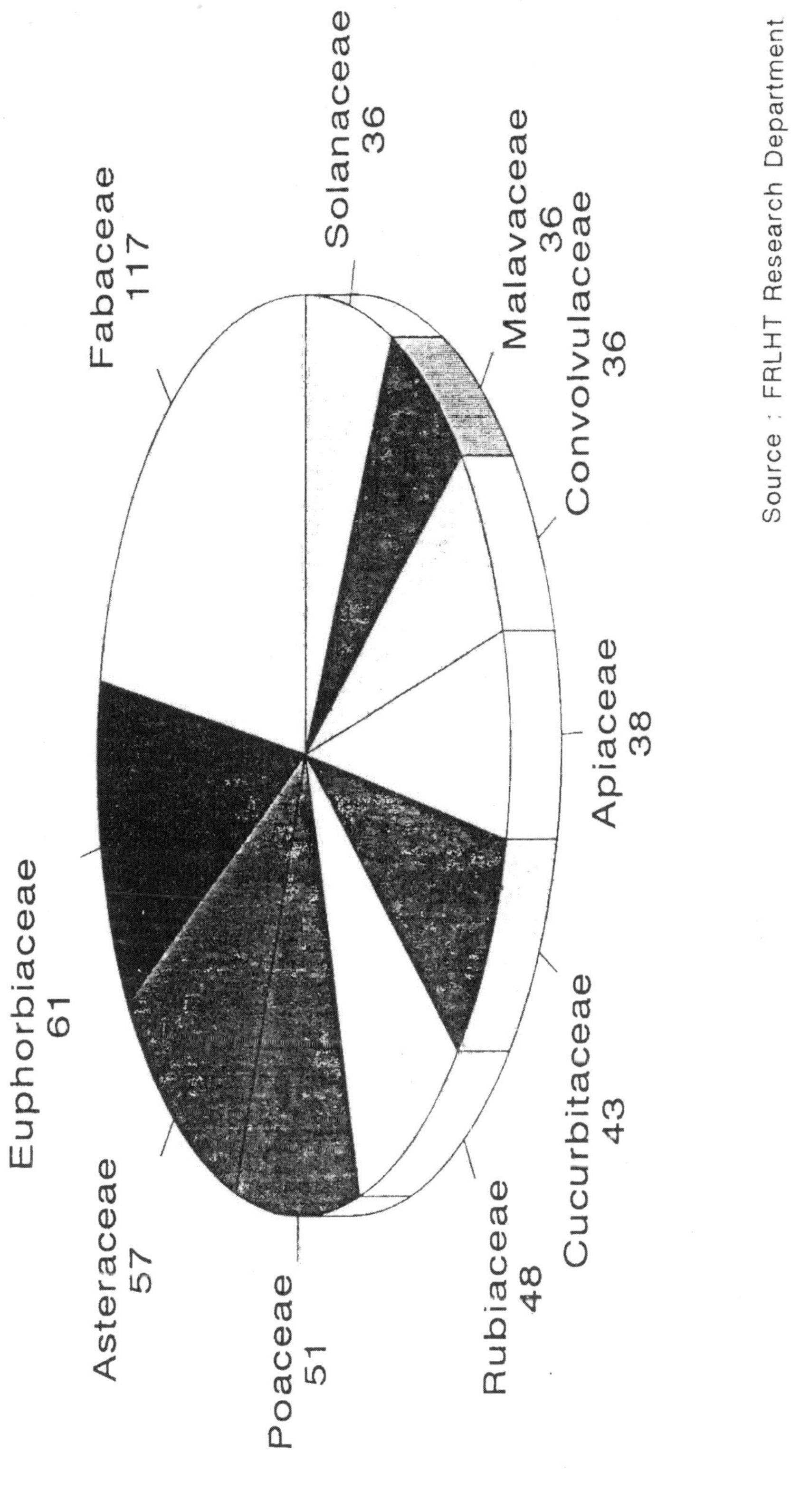

Figure 3: Distribution of Ayurvedic medicinal plants among the ten most represented families

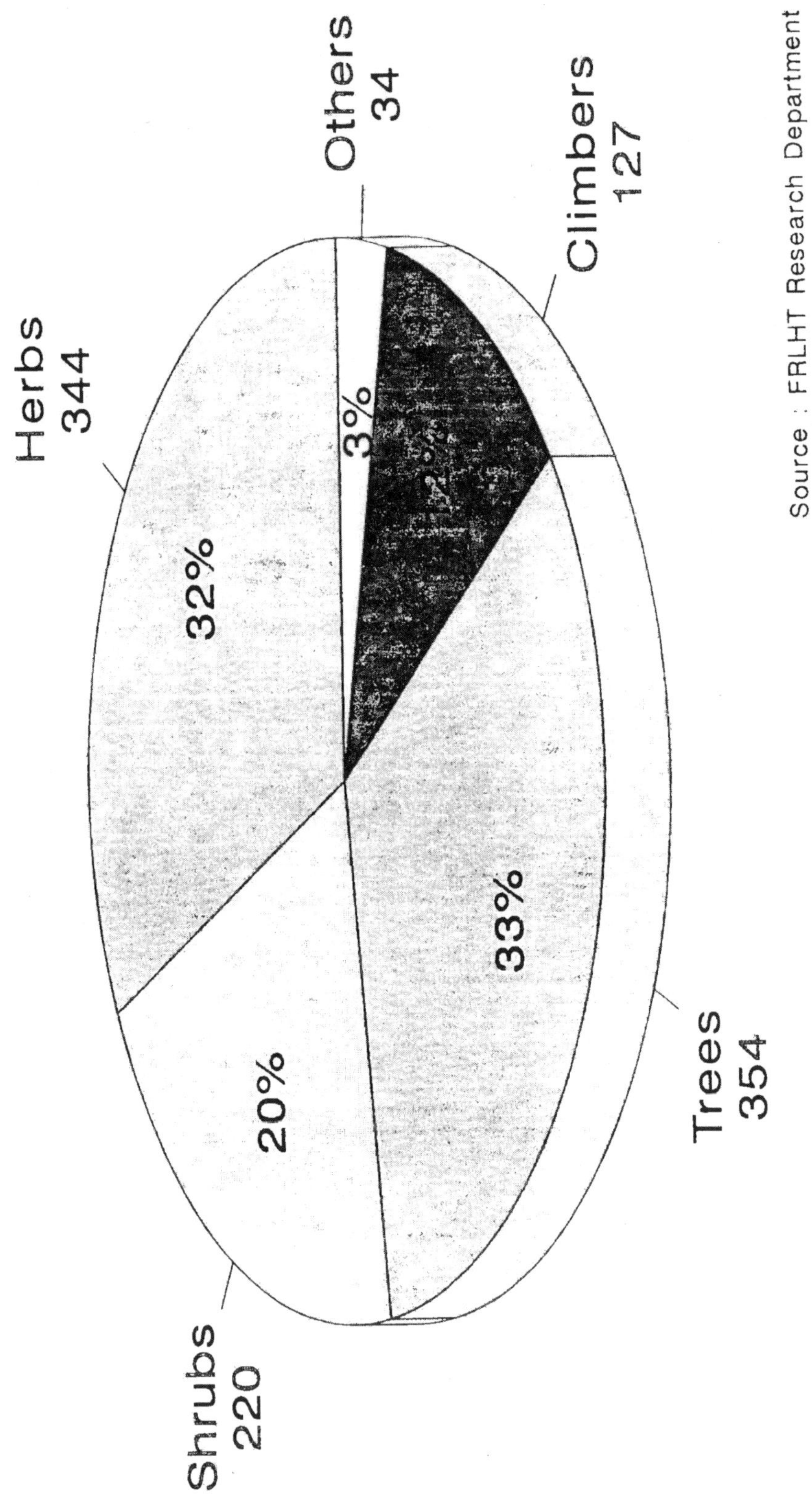

Figure 4: Diversity of medicinal plants of South India: habitat-wise analysis of 1079 species

The biodiversity loss is not only a threat to ecology of the planet but a more immediate threat to the livelihood security of rural communities.

Nature of traditional medicine in India

The biodiversity of medicinal plants is associated with a very rich cultural diversity related to India's traditional systems of medicine. Traditional Medicine as practised in India consists of two streams, viz. folk medicine and the codified systems of medicine.

Folk medicine

This is a diverse stream which is ecosystem and ethnic community specific. It is an oral tradition purely empirical in nature that exists in all rural communities throughout the length and breadth of India (Table 5).

Table 5. Types of carriers of village-based health traditions.*

Traditional carrier	Conditions treated	Numbers
Housewives and elders	Home remedies, food and nutrition-related	millions
Traditional birth attendants	Normal deliveries	700,000
Herbal healers	Common ailments	300,000
Bone setters	Orthopaedics	60,000
Visha vaidhyas (snake, scorpion , dog bite specialists)	Natural poisons	60,000
Other specialists	Eyes, skin, respiratory, dental, arthritis, mental diseases, gastro-intestinal, wounds, fistula, piles	1,000 in each area

* Figures bases on extrapolations from micro-studies by FRLHT Research Department.

One comes across many examples of the great depth and range of the folk tradition in unpublished reports on medical practices in different regions. For instance, in 1793, two medical officers of the East India Company - James Finlay and Thomas Cruso - reported on the practice of rhinoplasty by a potter's community in Pune district in the Madras Gazette (and later in 1794 in the London Gentleman's Magazine). It was this technical report that led to further developments in Britain of plastic surgery of the nose. To cite a current example, it is well known in south Karnataka that certain paralytic conditions can effectively be treated using 'Ankola' oil (In a place called Ankola in southern Karnataka, this treatment is administered by a tribal practitioner). Ankola is the name of a village; this particular herbal oil is part of its folk medical legacy. There is also the case, in Tamil Nadu state, of the so-called 'Coimbatore orthopaedic treatment' for straightening out a club foot by the combined use of a special herbal oil which softens the bony tissues and traditional forms of traction (Telungu Palayam Original Hospital in Coimbatore, Tamil Nadu, is a traditional orthopaedic centre where club foot and other outstanding orthopaedic procedures are practised). Yet another example is the use of the bitter aqueous extract of *Alstonia scholaris* bark by many rural communities at the start of monsoons, as a protection against malarial fevers.

Codified traditional medicine

Systems like Ayurveda, Unani, Siddha and the Tibetan system are expressions of this stream. The 'codified' stream consists of medical knowledge with sophisticated theoretical foundations expressed in thousands of regional manuscripts covering treatises on all branches of medicine and surgery. However, of an estimated 100,000 medical manuscripts lying in oriental libraries and private collections in India and abroad, less than one percent are available and in current use by students and teachers in Indian medical schools. The earliest Ayurvedic texts, the Susruta Samhita and Caraka Samhita, are believed to have been written between 1500 and 1000 BC. The main branches of Ayurveda are Kayacikitsa (General Medicine), Balacikitsa (paediatrics), Grahacikitsa (Psychiatry), Salakya Tantra (Ophthalmology and ENT), Salya Cikitsa (Surgery), Visa Cikista (Toxicology), Rasayana (Rejuvenation) and Vajikarana (reproductive health). Besides these, there are specialised treatises on a range of subjects including Pharmacy (Bhesaja Kalpana), Pharmacopoeia (Nighantu), Diagnostics (Nidana), Special diagnostic techniques like Pulse diagnosis (Nadi Cikista), Iatrochemistry (Rasasastra), Dietetics (Pathyapathya), Pharmacology (Dravyaguna) and Positive health and preventive medicine (Svastha Vrtta).

Today there are over 400,000 licensed registered practitioners of the codified stream practising in the towns and cities of India (Ministry of Health, 1991). They offer a wide range of treatments as shown in the examples listed in Table 6.

Unfortunately, despite the large presence of a "living bio-health culture" in villages throughout India, it receives marginalised policy and financial support from national and international agencies, either for conserving its bioresources or for maintaining its indigenous knowledge base. This is evidently due to the western ethnocentric bias in health policies around the globe (Bodeker, 1994).

Challenge facing the cultural heritage

Whereas the reasons for loss of plant diversity are well known, the reasons for loss of cultural diversity are much less understood. These are briefly outlined here as a detailed treatment of the issue is outside the scope of this article.

In the domain of knowledge, non-western medical systems like Ayurveda have so far failed to stake their claims to originality. Their epistemological foundations lie unexplored outside of their cultural worlds. The universal attributes of the indigenous knowledge systems remain unrecognised due to the marginalised political status of the southern societies and more mundanely due to the limitations of language and ethnicity.

A major problem that non-western societies have to contend with in any serious evaluation of their own indigenous knowledge systems, is the common claim of all western scientists and philosophers that, after all, science is one, universal and uniquely expressed in the western scientific paradigms. Thus, while it may be possible to conceive of alternative methodologies, theories and practices in other domains such as music, linguistics, logic, art and politics, there is no such possibility conceded with regard to alternative sciences.

Table 6. Examples of strength of codified stream.

Discipline	Nature of treatment or advice offered
Prenatal care	detailed diet and promotive herbs; behaviorial advice for healthy progeny and for all stages of foetal development
Obstetrics	reliable advice which can help in ease of delivery
Post -natal care	herbs that can raise the general immunity of the mother & child
Food & nutrition	advice on seasonal diets suited to different constitutions; advice on specific (therapeutic) diets for various ailments/disease stages; food values provided on a range of relevant parameters different from modern nutrition; advice on incompatible foods
Gynaecology	Safe herbal treatments for all typical ailments of women; better management of suspected infertility conditions
Respiratory disorders	Safe herbal treatments for entire range of respiratory disorders including asthamatic conditions & allergies
Skin disorders	Safe herbal treatments for wide range of skin conditions including diseases like Psoariasis and Erysipelas
GIT disorders	Safe herbal treatments for hyperacidity, ulcers & metabolic disorders
Cardiac diseases	herbal drugs for lowering chlorestrol, chronic angina and congenital heart diseases
Ophthalmology	Safe herbal treatments for intra-occular haemorrhage, diabetic retinopathy, paediatric myopia and a range of common eye diseases
Orthopaedics	management of compound factures with open wounds; management of polio; management of osteal deformities
Nervous & muscular disorders	herbal drugs for degenerative diseases in their early stages; hemiplegia, paraplegia, cereberal palsy etc.
Mental health	safe herbal drugs for anxiety neurosis, obsessions, hysteric manifestations, epilepsy etc.
Specific diseases	Herbal treatments for non-insulin-dependent diabetes, arthritis, hepatitis, rheumatic fevers, gall & kidney stone, ano-fistulas & haemorrhoids, promotive care of cancer and AIDS cases

The fact, however, is that different cultures have developed fundamentally different ways of perceiving and viewing nature and this in turn has given rise to different traditions of knowledge (See Fig. 5).

The chart in Fig. 5 depicts the differences in foundations, concepts and categories of Ayurveda and modern medicine. These differences should cause no surprise to anyone who is willing to accept the inevitable plurality of cultures.

Can traditional systems of medicine be explained in terms of modern medicine?

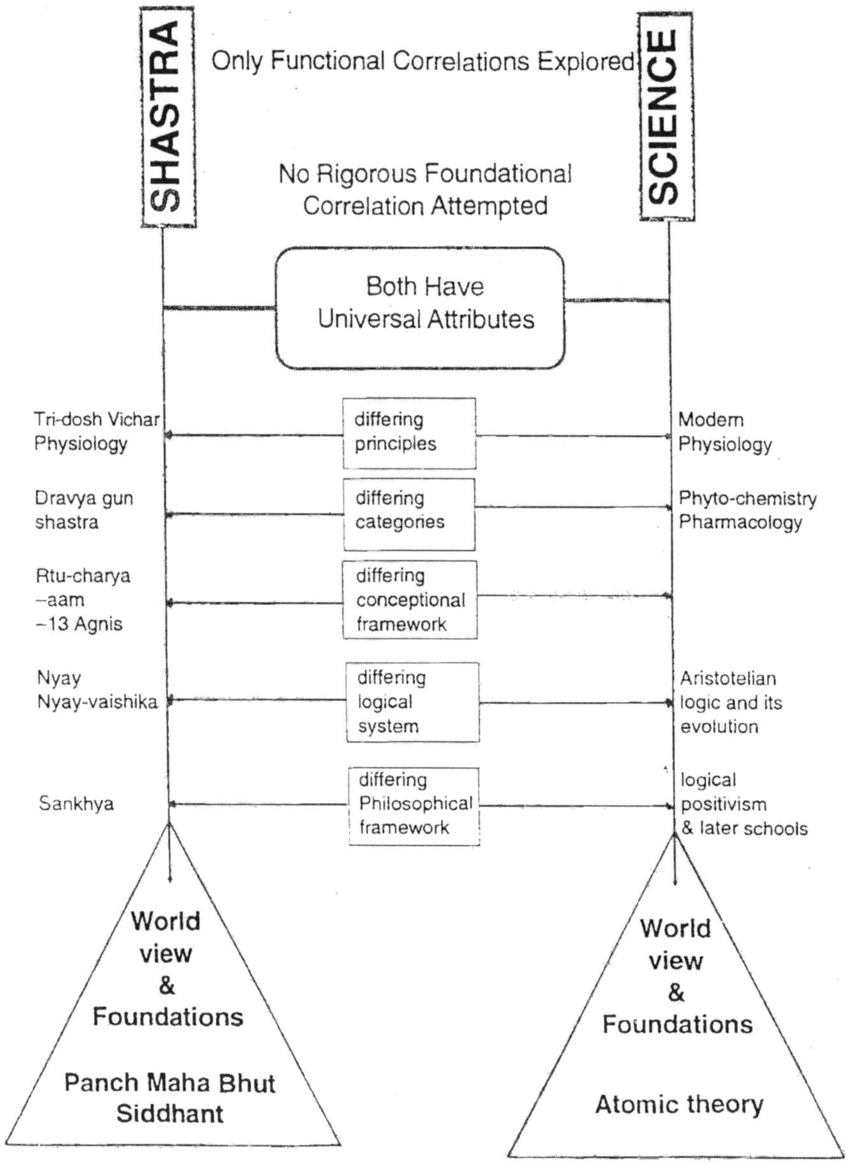

Figure 5: Epistemological foundations of Ayurveda and modern science

The comparative understanding between Ayurveda and modern medicine in fact has not progressed sufficiently to correlate diagnosis of the two systems of medicine or translate Ayurvedic pharmacology (Dravya gun shastra) in terms of modern pharmacological parameters or reduce Ayurvedic lines of treatment to satisfy Allopathic therapeutic logic.

Efficacy of disease management by Ayurvedic means and methods based on its own theories and monitored using modern parameters could form the basis for a dialogue between the two systems where the outcome would be in the form of *prima facie* evidence of success or failure in management but not a one-to-one correlation in diagnosis or a modern explanation of how and why of the traditional line of treatment.

The scope of this kind of comparative research designs from the modern medicine viewpoint will inevitably be limited. It will provide modern medicine only with some evidence of the efficacy or otherwise of Ayurvedic management. If modern medicine wants to apply the success of Ayurvedic treatment more widely based on the *prima facie* results, it will have to take the trouble to learn Ayurvedic principles and its diagnostic, pharmacological and treatment theories and procedures. The kind of comparative research outlined above will not, for instance, lead to any 'short-cut' ways to directly co-opt Ayurvedic drugs into the modern Materia Medica. This should be seen as a short-term loss. A pursuance of genuine dialogue with the traditional systems of medicine may pave the way for more meaningful long-term advances in world medicine that may broaden the scope of modern understanding of health and disease at more fundamental levels.

Conclusion

Conservation of medicinal plants in its biocultural perspective not only implies conservation of biodiversity but also places an equal emphasis on conservation of cultural diversity. The debilitating ecological consequences of monoculture in biological life are well known. The effects of promoting a monoculture in the civilisational context is only now being recognised.

References

Abdul Kareem 1995. *Inventory of Plants used in Indian Systems of Medicine*. FRLHT Research Report, Bangalore, India.

ADMA 1996. All India Ayurvedic Drug Manufacturers Association. Personal communication.

AICEP 1994. *Summary Report* of the All India Coordinated Ethno-biological Project (AICEP) of Ministry of Environment & Forests, Government of India.

Alvares, C. 1984. *Homo Faber*. New Delhi, India; Mentor Publications.

Anthropological Survey of India 1994. *People of India Project Report* for 1994.

Bodeker, G. 1994. Traditional health knowledge and public policy. *Nature and Resources* 30 (2): 5-16.

Darshan Shankar 1992. Indigenous health services. In: *State of India's Health*. Published by Voluntary Health Association of India.

Dharmpal 1983. *Indian Science and Technology in the 18th Century*. Hyderabad, India; Academy of Gandhian Studies.

Farnsworth, N. R. & Soejarto, D.D. 1991. Global importance of medicinal plants. In: Akerele, O, Heywood, V. & Synge, H. (eds) *Conservation of Medicinal Plants*. Cambridge, UK; Cambridge University Press.

Kulkarni, D.K. 1994. *Ethno-botanical Knowledge of the "Mahadev Koli Tribals" of Western Maharastra*. Ph.D. Thesis, Agarkar Research Institute, Pune, India.

LSPSS 1993. Micro-studies carried out by members of All India network of NGOs (LSPSS, Coimbatore) involved in the revitalisation of local health traditions.

Ministry of Health 1991. Statistics of Ministry of Health, Government of India, Report for 1991.

Palekar, R.P. 1995. *Studies on Medical Traditions of Thakur Tribals*. Karajat, Maharashtra, India; Academy of Development Science.

Sushrut Samhita (5th Edition) 1992. Varanasi, India; Chowkhamba Prakashana Publishers.

A biocultural medicinal plants conservation project in Sri Lanka

Lyn de Alwis
Principal Co-Ordinator and Project Executant
WWF Project 3320
30 Hotel Road, Mt. Lavinia
Sri Lanka
Tel: 94-1-712451 Fax: 94-1-573098

Abstract

Sri Lanka has a rich flora consisting of some 3,000 species of vascular plants, over a quarter of which are endemic. The number of species used in traditional medicine is estimated to be between 550 and 700. Deforestation for economic development and the increasing demand for medicinal plant material collected from the wild pose serious threats to its biodiversity. Efforts being made within the framework of the WWF Project 3320 aimed at conserving the country's biodiversity are summarised.

Introduction

Every society has developed a medical system for maintaining the health of its population. F.L. Dunn, writing in "Asian Medical Systems" (Leslie, 1977), defines a medical system as "the pattern of social institutions and cultural traditions that evolves from deliberate behaviour to enhance health". In modern parlance this means that an individual's life style affects the well being of others in the community. This comes out very clearly in the word *Ayurveda*, the traditional Indian system, for *Ayu* means life or living, and *Veda* means science or medicine, in other words, the science of living.

Ayurveda, which reached Sri Lanka perhaps 2,500 years ago, has much to do with living in harmony with one's environment. Here environment is viewed in its totality, the interdependence of the living elements of plants with the non-living, air (including sunlight), water and soil.

My childhood in a rural community naturally exposed me to Ayurvedic physicians, or who in those colonial days were, perhaps in a derogatory sense, referred to as "native doctors". Only when I grew up did I realise that the doctor's medicines were found in nature, raised in flower pots ("pot herbs"), e.g. coriander, Iriveriya (*Plectranthus*), ginger (*Zingiber*), or gathered from the vicinity (home gardens) e.g. *Adhathoda vasica*, bael fruit (*Aegle marmelos*) or from a piece of waste land nearby, e.g. *Calatropis*.

Our dependence on plants was brought home more forcefully when we realised we could subsist on what grew around us: Gotukola (*Centella asiatica*) leaves, spinach, water cress, and the leaves and flowers of *Sesbania grandiflora*, would be served up at lunch time while stir-fried *Amaranthus* varieties and different lentils enriched dinner, all garnished, of course, with fresh ginger, garlic and cumin seed.

Realisation came later that animals shared these same delectable items. Also that the wild counterparts of similar food plants formed the bulk of a herbivore's diet. Could it be that human beings evolved their medical systems by closely observing wild animals? These surmises have been amply proven by my over 40 years of observing and studying natural history in the wilds of Sri Lanka, India, Nepal, Malaysia, Thailand and Cambodia, and through association with the ethnic populations that dwell there.

The strong cultural appeal of Ayurveda was tenaciously preserved in Sri Lanka because of its links with Buddhism, commencing with the exhortations of Lord Buddha himself. Buddhist monks and through them the ancient monarchy, practised Ayurveda, established state hospitals, nurtured herbal gardens and miniature forests, and actively encouraged the people to stay healthy. Thus it is easy to understand how a strictly traditional form of medicine steadily evolved into a science. Other factors which had and still have a bearing on the peoples' dependence and reliance on Ayurveda are, the ready availability of plants with the required therapeutic properties or, if purchased, their comparatively low cost, and very importantly, the absence of any after effects, which in many allopathic medications are warned against by the manufactures of synthetic drugs.

Despite the introduction of allopathy and 450 years of Western colonialism, Ayurveda lived on in the hearts and minds of the people of Sri Lanka. It was only after the massive deforestation that followed foreign domination with concomitant rural and urban "development", that herbal medicines were dealt some body blows and became moribund. However, soon after independence in 1948 when ethnic cultures staged a come-back, there was naturally a resurgence in Ayurveda. Once more the State elevated it to the level of Alternative Medicine, re-established hospitals and clinics in every province of the island, opened training institutes for would-be practitioners and reinstated the village physician as an approved professional.

Unfortunately the same zeal was not applied to the need to propagate or grow medicinal plants following their disappearance from home gardens and what were once village or community forests. A sudden influx of collectors into deeper forests and their irresponsible and often ruthless exploitation of nature, began to take its toll on wild populations which soon became threatened with extinction. Serious depletion of biodiversity was looming large.

It was against this backdrop that a proposal to conserve the medicinal plants of Sri Lanka was submitted to the World-wide Fund for Nature (WWF) in 1984 making use of the latter's Plants Campaign. This proposal was quickly approved in 1985, and Project 3320 - The Conservation of Medicinal Plants in Sri Lanka - was entrusted to me under the aegis of the Ministry of Indigenous Medicine and Cultural Affairs, one year later.

The flora of Sri Lanka

Before describing the project, it is necessary to look at the remarkable species diversity of the country's flora in order to appreciate the importance of plants to its people in their everyday life. Recent studies in ethnobotany have revealed an astonishing grasp of plant identification among rural people and their knowledge of the therapeutic properties these plants developed over generations. This is another reason for present day conservationist to strive to preserve both the traditional system of medicine and the plants on which it depends for its continuity.

For a relatively small island, a little over 25,500 sq miles (65,000 sq km) in extent, its species diversity is impressive. It is generally accepted that this has been made possible because its geographical position, its mild yet variable climate, very interesting topography and soil profiles which create numerous ecological niches for the evolution of diverse biotic communities.

Eisenberg and McKay (1970), Muller-Dumbois and Sirisena (1967), and Fernando (1967), identify seven vegetational zones, indirectly determined by climate. These are:

A1: Monsoon scrub jungle, extreme North and North-West
A2: Monsoon scrub jungle, extreme South-East
B: Monsoon forest and grassland
C: Inter-monsoon forest
D1: Rain forest and grassland - below 914 m
D2: Rain forest and grassland - 914m to 1524 m
D3: Rain forest & Grassland - above 1524 m

Despite manipulation of the environment by man over a period of some 2,500 years, Sri Lanka still has over 3,000 indigenous species of vascular plants of which about 850 (or over 25%) are endemic. In addition, there are possibly 70 early introductions, now naturalised, which have become economically important. The 3,000 species belong to 1,065 genera in 171 families. Of the 75% non-endemic indigenous species, about 65% have affinities with Indian & Himalayan forms, while the balance have come from Malaysian, African and Australian regions (Abeywickrema, 1956, 1959). Coupled with about 850 species of terrestrial vertebrates, this scenario presents excellent biological diversity.

Estimates made for the number of indigenous plant species used in medicine vary between reports. Abeywickrema (1979) puts the figure at "nearly 700" while Ekanayake (1981) lists 550. Both include about 35 species of naturalised exotics.

However, it is interesting to observe that of the indigenous plants common to Sri Lanka and India, about 305 find a place in traditional medicine. But as stated earlier, about 25% of Sri Lanka's flora is endemic, and only 3-4% of them have made their way into the local pharmacopoeias. The significance of this is two-fold: firstly that the local practitioners have faithfully followed the original system, and secondly and more importantly that at least another 20% of Sri Lanka's flora await study and research vis-à-vis the country's quest for more and perhaps better drugs.

The geographical distribution of the 550 species listed by Ekanayake (1981) is given in Table 1.

Table 1. Geographical distribution of indigenous medicinal plants of Sri Lanka (Ekanayake, 1981).

Biogeographical region	Number of species
Low country Wet zone	108
Low country Wet & Montane zone	40
Dry zone	148
Dry zone and Wet zone	189
Montane zone	25
Arid zone	2
Arid and Dry zone	7
Present in all regions	31
Total	550

It must be noted that Ekanayake has employed a slightly different zonal classification from the 7 zones described earlier. Be that as it may, the species distribution over a wide area tends towards an excellent gene pool which, if carefully protected, augurs well for the future.

Threats to biological diversity

Besides the almost inexorable removal of forest cover in the name of "economic development", in Sri Lanka medicinal plants are threatened in several other ways:

- the resurgence of traditional medicine in post-independence Sri Lanka,
- the concomitant demand for plant material to treat patients in the hospitals that are mushrooming throughout the country,
- the over-exploitation of natural plant populations to meet this demand,
- the waste of material due to erratic harvesting, poor storage and lack of proper marketing and transportation.

The number of Ayurvedic hospitals has increased sharply from less than 15 to 42 within 10 years causing havoc in the supply channels. Although Government and non-Government organisations have launched nurseries and herbal gardens in numerous school compounds, Buddhist temple lands and even on private property, the net production cannot meet the demand. This is mostly due to poor horticultural practices and lack of planting material because propagation of most medicinal plants was a neglected art.

The tendency still is for collection from the wild, often on a scale detrimental to the viability of populations. This is because fresh plants fetch very low prices compelling vendors to sell in bulk, e.g. 200 plants of the herb *Munronia pumila* an almost universal ingredient in many prescriptions, are uprooted to produce 1 kg of material. A collector will need about 200 plants (Rs 500.00 at 25 cents a plant) to make his expedition up and down rocky terrain worthwhile. This might mean the denudation of the whole microhabitat of this endemic species.

Again taking *Munronia* as an example, it is the dried plant that is used in medicine and if the drying has been insufficient, the whole consignment will be attacked by fungus and rejected by the market. Such wastage is a common feature in this trade and seriously endangers the species being exploited.

The project 3320

Project 3320 listed the following objectives:

- To advise the government on the need to protect medicinal plants in their natural habitats and to declare suitable areas as National Reserves for use on a sustainable basis.
- To conduct surveys of selected geographical zones to prepare checklist of plants correctly identified, and to assess population densities in order to determine threats to survival.
- To identify threatened species in order to propagate them using modern methods (e.g. tissue culture) in island-wide nurseries and reintroduce them into their natural habitats if and when necessary.
- To assist the Government in framing appropriate laws to ensure protection and to control commercial exploitation of important species.
- To assist the Government in preparing educational and publicity programmes to promote awareness and thus facilitate long-term conservation activities.
- To examine the cultural sites mentioned in ancient texts as having had herbal gardens with a view to revitalising them.

The Project was launched in June 1986.

A large number of organisations and many interested individuals were co-opted into an Advisory Committee from which, later, a Co-ordinating Committee was formed, each member charged with an activity which would realise the objectives of the Project. Thus, the Universities of Sri Jayawardenepura and Ruhuna, the Natural Resources Energy & Science Authority (NARESA), the Bandarnaike Memorial Ayurvedic Research Institute (MBRAI), the Royal Botanic Gardens, the Conservator of Forests and the Director of Wildlife Conservation each had a part to play.

In the beginning there were some problems which arose mostly from participants running away with the idea that the Projects' principal objective was the development of Ayurveda. It took a lot of doing to steer the Project on its main axis of conserving plants and their habitats for the future.

In 1990, therefore, the Project was reviewed with the help of Dr. Alan Hamilton, the WWF Plants Conservation Officer, under whose overall direction the project was functioning. It was decided at that time to concentrate on two significant goals: the protection of representative (natural) sites for genetic reserves and the cultivation of species in decline from wild sources.

Accordingly six new components were identified to achieve these goals. They are:

1. The establishment of a database to collate all available information and future findings in relation to the whole subject of medicinal plant conservation. The distribution and population density of species which resulted from field surveys occupy an important place in the database.

2. A market survey to determine present use and how such usage affects wild populations.

3. Field surveys covering all the major biogeographical zones.

4. Chemotaxonomic studies on medicinal plants to verify the therapeutic properties of different populations of one species and to determine the levels of genetic variability.

5. Legislation to control over-exploitation for local use as well as for export to pharmaceutical companies abroad.

6. Declaration of Special Natural Reserves for *in situ* conservation.

The results of components 2, 3 and 4 above provide the scientific and statistical information, hitherto seriously lacking, required to formulate conservation policy.

The market surveys revealed that ruthless extraction of fragile species from the wild was more widespread and destructive than previously thought. Nine species have been brought into a country list of endangered species for the protection of which legal provision is urgently required.

The scientific systematic surveys of representative natural sites in all the geographical zones have confirmed that the picture is not so rosy anymore. Practitioners even in rural areas complain of extirpation of certain species from their locality, notably species used in the treatment of fractures and of snake bite.

The re-survey of the hitherto jealously guarded cultural sites showed alarming depletion of immensely valuable species.

Chemotaxonomic studies have shown different genetic composition from different populations. For maintaining genetic diversity, it is essential to preserve natural populations wherever they occur, as gene banks.

A natural response to the unavailability of local herb species is to cultivate them or to introduce substitutes or, as a last resort, to import them. Cultivation has its limitations. Agronomic studies have already shown that the therapeutic value of cultivated species undergoes change with intensive cultivation practices. There have to be infusions from wild species if the therapeutic value of a medicinal herb is to be sustained. Other experiments carried out in the Botany department of the University of Matara showed that the application of agrochemicals did not directly or necessarily improve growth as occurs in other crops.

All these findings point to one goal: that of preserving species in their natural habitats.

Therefore, Project 3320 today is marching towards what could be identified as its most important goal - that of preserving biological diversity through the protection of natural habitats which support sizeable populations of either widely exploited species or those whose populations have reached critical levels. The work done so far under the Project as set out in the preceding paragraphs underscores the need for *in situ* conservation, providing the scientific data, the methodology and justification for establishing natural reserves.

Cultural heritage

According to the epic Asian story, the *Ramayana,* King Rama's beloved brother Lakshman lay gravely ill and the physician attending on him had prescribed medicines from herbs found only in the deep forests of the Himalayas. Rama therefore summoned Hanuman, the monkey-god, to fetch these herbs. Not being able to identify the herbs, Hanuman did the next best thing - he decided to carry back a piece of the forest itself. It is believed that while crossing over from the Himalayas to Lanka chunks of the forest had fallen along the way and that places like Ritigala (and Sigiriya), Dolukande in the north-west of the island and Rumassala in the south where medicinal herbs abound even today, mark some of these spots.

Even before Project 3320 was conceived, the government had decided to declare several cultural and historical sites as specially protected areas. Besides those already mentioned, Nilgala in the East-Central part of the country, Dolukande in the North-West, Rumassala in the South, and Singharaja in the West had also been earmarked. Subsequently Sigiriya and Ritigala in the North-Central Province, which are archaeological sites of great importance, were added on.

Our surveys of these sites under Project 3320 confirmed that these places were indeed very rich in medicinal plants in a natural state. Some of them like Dolukande and Rumassala had been extensively harvested and some species had reached critical levels. Dolukande has a total of 115 species while Rumassala recorded some 75. And what is more, these sites are jealously guarded by the incumbent Buddhist monks who look after the shrines at these sites. Clearly, therefore, all these sites had to be integrated into any overall plan for conservation of biological diversity and held in trust for posterity. WWF involvement at Sigiriya is a role model for integrating *ex situ, in situ* and cultural conservation. There, a 1-ha nursery has been progressively developed into a centre for both distributing plants to villagers and for reintroducing plants which have been extirpated. Sigiriya being a premier archaeological site for conservation under the UNESCO-aided Cultural Triangle, is the ideal location to showcase this new thinking. The herbal garden is now being extended into the adjacent forest to form a 10-acre *in situ* conservation site. Sigiriya is also redolent with ethnobotanical relationships which are being fully investigated only now. The herbal garden will soon be of educational value when its gates will be opened to school-children and members of the public who wish to study medicinal plants.

The present guardians of our Protected Areas as defined by IUCN, are the Forest Department and the Department of Wildlife Conservation. There are some 450 such Protected Natural Areas in the country and what better network could there be for the demarcation of Special Reserves for medicinal plants within some of them? The Protected Areas comprise Forest Reserves and Proposed Forest Reserves, National Parks, Sanctuaries and similar reserves for Wildlife, Wetlands, and Man and Biosphere (MAB) reserves.

The time is now opportune to go into partnership with the Forest Department for they are in the process of surveying selected sites for a National Conservation Register. Since these surveys concentrated only on trees of economic value, medicinal plants had been missed out. Now through discussion we have persuaded them to include herbs identified with the help of local Ayurvedic Practitioners, medicinal plant collectors and physicians from the nearest Ayurvedic Hospital. The Senior Scientist of the BMARI and Curator of the National Herbarium are also being consulted.

The Forest Department has identified 9 sites which will receive special protection under IUCN's Biological Diversity Programme. At least 5 of them have already been identified as being suitable for the protection of medicinal plant species and habitats. They are: Nilgala, Dolukande and Rumassala, already mentioned above, and Kiribathgoda and Rajawaka (Bellangala) in the Ratnapura District in the Wet Zone and the Intermediate Zone of the country.

All these sites have been established as possessing tremendous species diversity and they justify selection as Special Reserves. Nilgala, in particular, which is species rich today, is believed to have been given protection by the Sinhala kings in the past.

The Forest Department has given high priority to the declaration of the Rajawaka Proposed Forest Reserve as a Special Medicinal Plants Reserve. Besides its unusual floristics akin to that of Nilgala with a climax community of *Pterocarpus marsupium, Phyllanthus emblica, Terminalia belerica and T. chebula,* Rajawaka as its name implies, was the preserves of royalty (Royal Park) in ancient Sri Lanka. Today it still remains an important source of medicinal trees and plants, and is much sought after by the people in times of illness. Therefore, any form of protection will not impinge on the rights of villagers to collect material. Indeed, the Forest Department actually wishes to include participatory management by the people.

Project 3320 will be associated in the unique event of the declaration of Sri Lanka's first-ever Special Natural Reserves for medicinal plants in the following manner:

- Site selection: Since the concept of *in situ* conservation is to protect viable populations, each site will be a minimum of 100 ha. This size will facilitate monitoring of changes in the population as and when plants are utilized by local villagers. In certain cases the size will be much larger, particularly if plant density is thin on the ground or if there already is protection under one of the state ordinances, for example, relating to Forest, Wildlife or Archaeology.
- Species to be protected: Because neither the Forest Department nor the Wildlife Conservation Department has a history of medicinal herb protection, Project 3320 will

provide persons to identify the species and populations which preponderate in a selected site.

Preparation of a Management Plan: New management approaches need to be developed for the selected site and incorporated into the overall Management Plan of, say, the Forest Reserve, Wildlife National Park or Archaeological Site. This will include preparation of plant lists, their density, seasonal fluctuation, usage patterns, etc. The Management Plan will try to protect the whole habitat and entire populations.

- The widest representation of bio-geographical zones will be surveyed and recommended for inclusion in the programme.
- Assisting the Government agency concerned in designing projects which involve rural peoples and obtain their participation in safeguarding this natural resource.
- Providing finances for such items as: physical demarcation where feasible, e.g. coloured fencing posts where the site is small, allowances to individuals, staff and others involved in the protection, fuel for patrolling by vehicles where the site is large.

Concurrently there will be educational and awareness programmes for the beneficiaries to appreciate the usefulness of preserving species and biological diversity for their future well being.

The first site which is a Proposed Forest Reserve known as Rajawaka or Bellangala has been selected and preliminary work started. This is presently a source of medicinal plants for a cluster of villages. If not properly managed, it may not remain a sustainable resource for much longer.

Project 3320 has been successful in bringing to light the exact situation with regard to the danger that awaits biological diversity in the realm of medicinal plants. The constraints identified are timely and the Government is being advised to initiate the actions proposed before it is too late.

Conclusion

With these scientific and cultural initiatives, it is hoped that Project 3320 will mark the beginning of a new approach to ensuring continuity of a medical science through the preservation of the natural resources on which it depends. This Project can be emulated as a model for medicinal plant conservation in both biodiversity and biocultural contexts.

Utilization and conservation of medicinal plants in China
with special reference to *Atractylodes lancea*

Shan-An He and Ning Sheng
Jiangsu Institute of Botany
Nanjing Botanical Garden, Mem. Sun Yat-Sen
P.O. Box 1435 Nanjing
Jiangsu 210014
Peoples' Republic of China

Abstract

Approximately 1,000 plant species are commonly used in Chinese medicinal preparations. More than three-quarters of these are collected from the wild. The demand for medicinal plant material has grown at an annual rate of 9% over the past two decades. The threat posed by overexploitation and the measures which need to taken for the conservation and cultivation of medicinal plants are highlighted using *Atracylodes lancea* as an example.

Introduction

Medical and pharmaceutical traditions of China have evolved over the centuries as essential parts of its civilization and are widely recognized today as representing its rich cultural and scientific heritage. As this medical knowledge and expertise were built on a land endowed with an abundance of varied flora, it is not surprising that medicinal plants play a central role in Chinese medicine and the country's achievement in the utilization of its native plants in health care delivery has been admired and acknowedged throughout the world.

According to a recent study (He and Cheng, 1990), the total number of species of medicinal plants used in different parts of the country add up to over ten thousand. According to a Chinese proverb, "Every plant is a medicinal herb."

Present status of utilization of medicinal plants in china

The official *Pharmacopoeia of People's Republic of China* lists 709 different drugs. Among these, only a little more than 40 items are animal and mineral products. Others are all derived from plant material. Plant material accounts for more than 80% of the drugs sold on the market. Approximately 1000 species of plants are now commonly used in Chinese medicine and about half of these are considered as the main medicinal plants which are in particularly common use. Material from these 1,000 species is harvested and marketed extensively. Medicinal plants are distributed over a wide geographic area ranging from 50°N (Helongjiang province) to 10°N (Hainan province) and from 80°E to 130°E.

The government has introduced a series of laws, regulations and rules to provide guidelines for and to control the collection, cultivation, production, certification, registration and marketing of medicinal plants in order to promote the development of Chinese medicines in the most appropriate manner and to protect public health and safety.

If we consider the most common ailments affecting wide sections of the population, *viz*. cancer, cardiovascular diseases, hepatitis, influenza and various kinds of fevers, then the most popularly used medicinal plants are either those in the group used for increasing the person's immunity and resistance to diseases, e.g. *Panax notoginseng, Panax quinquefolium, Cordyceps sinensis, Eucommia ulmoides, Gastrodia elata, Ganoderma lucidum* etc. or are among other medicinal plants used for specific conditions, e.g. *Dioscorea* spp., *Salvia miltiorrhiza, Astragalus membranaceus* var. *mongholicus, Glycyrrhiza uralensis and Bupleurum chinense.*

It should be remembered, however, that prescriptions in the Chinese system of medicine nearly always consist of material from several different plants.

Trends in the utilization of medicinal plants

Whereas both traditional Chinese medicine and western medicine form part of today's health care system in China, the former is more popular among the country's population at large. The state offers assistance and support to the cultivation of medicinal plants and, at the same time, promotes the development of an integrated health care delivery system which combines traditional Chinese medicine with modern western medicine. Most large hospitals offer treatment based on both systems and it is very common for patients to receive both Chinese medicines and western medicines for their illness. Sometimes they take both kinds of medicines at the same time and sometimes alternatively.

People suffering from ailments for which there is no satisfactory treatment in western medicine, no matter whether they live in rural areas or in cities, always look for alternatives based on traditional Chinese medicine. Many studies comparing the relative efficacies of Chinese and western medicines for a range of conditions, both chronic and acute, have established the superiority of the former (NABCMD, 1989). Examples of chronic conditions include chronic anaemia, lupus erythematosus, stomach cancer and ABO haemolytic disease of new-born babies. Examples of acute conditions include mortality from haemorrhagic fever caused by wild mouse, myocardial infarction, pancreatitis, and cholangitis.

Discovery of the anti-malarial drug Qinghaosu from *Artemisia annua* and the medicine for hepatitis derived from *Swertia milensis* have further proved the future potential of Chinese medicinal plants. Plants used in Chinese traditional medicine which have shown promise as potential sources of anticancer and anti-HIV compounds include *Glycyrrhiza uralensis, Ligusticum chuanxiong, Astragalus membranaceus* var. *mongholicus, Schisandra chinensis , Atractylodes lancea, Acanthopanax senticosus, Panax ginseng, Lithospermum erythrorrhizon, Senecio scandens* and *Coptis chinensis* (Zhun, 1991).

During the period from 1979 to 1990, forty-two new Chinese medicinal preparations appeared on the market (Song, 1992). Among them 11 are for cardiac diseases, five for cancer and six for ailments of the digestive system (Huang, 1990). The green movement and the current trend of "coming back to the nature" have led to a renewed interest in traditional medicinal plants. A new aspect, namely the use of fresh medicinal plant material, is worth mentioning. Recent studies carried out at the Jiangsu Institute of Botany (Nanjing Botanical Garden, Mem. Sun Yat-Sen) on the efficacy of fresh herbs in treatment for the skin diseases, herpes, caused by viruses. A Chinese medicine named "Eliherpes" has proved particularly effective in the treatment of herpes zoster, herpes simplex and sexual herpes. In a clinical trial involving more than 200 patients, it was found to be effective in 94.36% of the cases. The medicine is inexpensive, safe to use and easy to administer. It provides quick pain relief and rapid healing without sequelae. This new approach using fresh herbs has been developed and applied for treating patients in some hospitals in Nanjing city already.

Overexploitation of natural resources and the necessity for conservation and cultivation of medicinal plants

Until now, the major part of plant material used in Chinese medicines has originated from wild sources. Among the 1,000 commonly used medicinal plants, 80% in terms of number species and 60% in terms of total quantity have come from wild sources. Overexploitation is a problem common to all medicinal plants. For most species, the natural reserves are exhausted within 10 to 20 years of collection. For some species the supplies from the wild last only for three or four years, after which no more commercial production is possible. It should be noted that the loss of genetic variation within a given species is usually much more serious and occurs much earlier than the total extinction of the species itself. For example, the content of diosgenin in *Dioscorea zingiberensis* collected during expeditions in the 1950s averaged only 7% whereas the maximum recorded was about 17%. In material collected during the 1980s the content was reduced to such an extent that even 4% was considered as high. When the medicine using *Swertia milensis* was developed for the treatment of hepatitis, a shortage in the supply of plant material appeared within three to four years (Wang, 1992).

In the past, the distribution of *Glycyrrhiza uralensis* was mainly concentrated in Inner Mongolia. In the 1950s *G. uralensis* grew over an area of 1.2 million ha. By 1981 this was reduced to only 330 thousand ha. The center of western growing area had therefore moved to the Xinjiang autonomous region (Yuan, Wang and Lu, 1992). The situation is not any better in the eastern growing area either. In the 1960s the plain of Nenjiang river was famous for its *G. uralensis* population. Twenty years later there were no bushes with any commercial value left in this area. Preliminary statistics indicate that approximately 6,000 tons of *G. uralensis* are exported annually and the domestic consumption amounts to several thousand tons (Fu and Du, 1987).

A similar situation of shortage has also been observed for the following species: *Cistanche deserticola, Cordyceps sinensis, Asarum heterotropoides* var. *mandshuricum, Phellodendron chinense, Eucommia ulmoides, Magnolia officinalis, Gastrodia elata, Ephedra sinica, Acanthopanax senticosus, Bupleurum chinense, Paris polyphylla, Atractylodes lancea* and *Notopterygium incisum.*

The depletion of resources has accelerated with increasing demand for Chinese medicinal preparations both at home and abroad. Since 1979 the demand has increased at a rate of 9% per year. In 1987 the total production had reached 650 thousands tons (Chinese Yearbook of Pharmacology, 1987). There are altogether more than 600 industrial plants producing over 4,000 composite drugs in 40 different formulations. In 1978 the total value was RMB 3.6 billion. In 1990, the total quantity was 20 thousand tons and the total value RMB 5.5 billion. By 1992, this had increased to RMB 11 billion. Chinese medicinal preparations are exported to more than 100 countries and the total value of exports is in the region of 100-200 million U.S. dollars (Li, 1992).

The only solution to this rapid exhaustion of resources is cultivation. Since the 1980s there has been a rapid increase in the area cultivated with medicinal plants. In 1984 the total land area devoted to medicinal plant cultivation was 380 thousand ha which is about 161% of that in 1981.

At present there are more than 250 species of medicinal plants being commercially cultivated. Among them about 60 species have performed particulary well under cultivation (Institute of Medicinal Plant Development, 1991). The main crops cultivated are as follows: *Gastrodia elata, Panax ginseng, Panax notoginseng, Cordyceps sinensis, Coptis chinensis, Eucommia ulmoides, Glycyrrhiza uralensis, Fritillaria cirrhosa, Fritillaria thunbergii, Astragalus membranaceus* var. *mongholicus, Asarum heterotropoides* var. *mandshuricum, Schisandra chinensis, Platycodon grandiflorum, Pinellia ternata, Polygonum multiflorum, Macrocarpium officinale, Dendrobium nobile, Gynostemma pentaphyllum, Saposhnikovia divaricata, Gentiana manshurica, Salvia miltiorrhiza, Anemarrhena asphodeloides, Bupleurum chinense, Corydalis turtschaninovii* f. *yanhusuo, Crocus sativus, Belamcanda chinensis* and *Cimicifuga foetida*.

Concurrently with these developments in the cultivation of Chinese medicinal plants, many exotic medicinal plants have been introduced and brought under cultivation. About 30 introduced species have successfully been grown during the past 30 years. The main among these are as follows: *Eugenia aromatica, Scaphium lychnophorum, Amomum compactum, Strychnos wallichiana, Styrax tonkinensis, Silybum marianum, Panax quinquefolium, Atropa belladonna* and *Digitalis lanata*.

Active research is being carried out on various aspects of cultivation and processing of a wide range of medicinal plants. Examples include: rapid propagation of *Siraitia grosvenorii* and *Aloe vera* var. *chinensis*; the use of fermentation technology for the processing of *Cordyceps sinensis, Ganoderma lucidum* and *Armillaria mellea*; tissue culture for the production of active principles of *Panax ginseng, Panax notoginseng, Ligusticum chuanxiong, Glycyrrhiza uralensis, Panax quinquefolium, Lithospermum erythrorrhizon, Hyoscyamus niger, Corydalis turtschaninovii* f. *yanhusuo*; and imporoving cultural practices for higher yields and better quality of *Eucommia ulmoides, Coptis chinensis, Magnolia officinalis, Lonicera japonica* and *Tripterygium wilfordii*. (NABCMD, 1989; Peng and Xiao, 1993).

In addition to the species under cultivation, approximately 2,000 species of exotic medicinal plants are currently maintained in Chinese botanical gardens.

A case study: *Atractylodes lancea*

Exhaustion of resources

A. lancea is an example of species of which the natural population size has decreased seriously as as a result of overcollection. In semi-cultivated species, the loss of genetic variability occurs very rapidly and can reach serious levels even in the absence of any significant decrease in the total number of individuals. The conservation of a medicinal plant species with a wide range of genetic diversity is therefore even more difficult than that of rare and endangered species with a small number of individuals. As cultivation has a very strong influence on the erosion of genetic variability, for many semi-cultivated medicinal plants, in spite of the apparent stability in their total population size, conservation measures are required as urgently as for rare and endangered species.

Although *A. lancea* is widely distributed in central China, the traditional, high quality medicinal material called *Mao-Cangzhu* comes from the Maoshan mountains. This plant is mainly used for the treatment of indigestion and stomach disorders. The highest recorded production of this crude drug in Jiangsu province was 6.6 tons per year. But in 1983 the annual production was only 1.2 tons. Based on the production figures for *A. lancea* in five counties of Jiangsu province, *viz.* Juroug, Jintan, Lishui, Liyang and Gaochun, the highest production was recorded in the 1950s. The figures for the 1980s were much lower than those for the 1960s and 1970s. Resources of *A. lancea* were seriously being depleted in all five counties in Jiangsu. The data indicate a sharp reduction in deposits as soon as commercial collecting activities began. The existing resources would only last for 10-20 years if no steps are taken towards conservation. The slow growth rate of the species is an important reason for such a rapid depletion. Experiments to measure growth rates have shown that the rhizome grows only to twice its original size in any given year. Protection and cultivaiton are therefore absolutely essential for *A. lancea* (He *et al.*, 1993).

Determination of genetic variation

A knowledge of genetic variation is essential for conservation purposes as well as for selecting the appropriate planting material to use in agronomic work aimed at improving production under cultivation.

Although the Maoshan area is the famous region for the Cangzhu variety of *A. lancea*, the species is distributed over a wide area including Jiangsu, Zhejiang, Shandong, Anhui, Hubei and Sichuan provinces. Based on the data for Jiangsu, Anhui and Hubei provinces, it grows at altitudes from 60 to 1,000 m above mean sea level. The sites investigated have a relatively similar climatic pattern, except for precipitation which varied between sites from 850 to 1,560 mm per year. Soils are mostly acidic, about pH 5, and occasionally alkaline, pH 7.5, The rocks are mostly granite and quartzite, but also limestone in places. High density distributions of Cangzhu *A. lancea* are usually found only on the north facing slopes.

Morphological differences have been observed between plants growing under different ecological conditions. For verifying the morphological differences which are genuinely due to genetic factors, plant samples were collected and cultivated in the Nanjing Botanical Garden experimental plots. Collections from various designated sites were propagated vegetatively. Plants of different provenances had different leaf shapes (Fig.1) and it has been confirmed that these are due to real genetic variation among them.

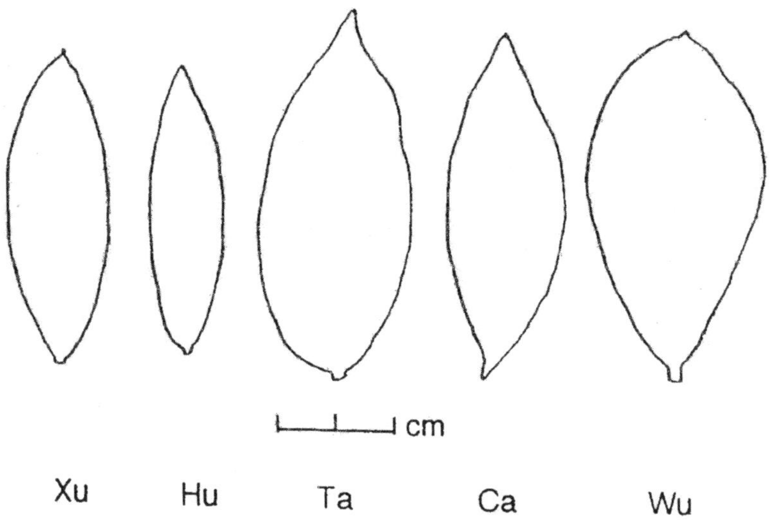

Figure 1: Leaf shapes of *Atractylodes lancea* according to different provenances in China

Morphological information alone is not sufficient for making decisions concerning the choice of appropriate provenances for conservation or cultivation. For these purposes, it is also essential to know the active principle content of the plant material. Analyses of the major active constituents of *A. lancea* showed that not only plants growing in different geographic areas with different morphological characteristics could have different chemical constituents but also plants with similar morphological features and growing on the same site may have different contents of chemical constituents. For example, analyses carried out on 144 samples collected from four sites in Jiangsu province with similar morphological features indicated that there were at least two variations with respect to the presence or absence of various chemical constituents (Table 1).

Table 1. Variations in chemical composition of *Atractylodes lancea*

Variation	Number of samples	Percentage of total population	Presence (+) or absence (-) of constituents			
			Atractylon	Hinesol	Eudesmol	Atractylodin
Type 1	27	19	+	+	+	+
Type 2	73	51	+	-	-	+
Others	44	30	Outside the above types			
Total	144	100				

For conservation we may obtain specimens exhibiting different characteristics including morphological and chemical variations, and keep them in the collection. But for the choice of material for cultivation, more studies need to be carried out on the clinical effectiveness of the different provenances, especially based on their chemical composition. This kind of research usually takes a relatively long time. This example illustrates the complexity of the various issues involved in the conservation and cultivation of medicinal plants.

References

Chinese Year Book of Pharmacology. 1987. Chinese Medicines: A general report on 9 years' reform of Chinese medicines and Scientific research. Beijing, China; Public Health Press. pp. 166-167.

Fu, K.Z. & Du, Y. X. 1987. A proposal for the establishment of *Glycyrrhiza* plantations for commercial production in north-eastern China. *Journal of Chinese Medicines* 12: (5) 3-5.

He, S. A. & Cheng, Z. M. 1991. The role of Chinese botanical gardens in conservation of medicinal plants. In: Akerele, O., Heywood, V. & Synge, H. (eds) *Conservation of Medicinal Plants*. Cambridge; UK; Cambridge University Press. pp. 229-237.

He, S. A. *et al.* 1993. The conservation and utilization of *Atractylodes lancea* (Thunb.) DC. *Journal of Plant Resources and Environment* 2: (1) 1-6.

Huang, T.K. 1990. New Chinese medicines in 1990. *Medical and Pharmaceutical Information* 5: 53.

Institute of Medicinal Plant Development. 1991. *Cultivation of Chinese Medicinal Plants*. Beijing, China; Agricultural Press. 1375 pp.

Li, J.K. 1992. To speed the steps of preparing Chinese medicines for the world. *Chinese Prepared Medicines* 14: (9) 42-43.

National Adiministrative Burean of Chinese Medicial and Drugs. 1989. *Scientific and Technical Achievements of Chinese Medicine during 1949-1989*. Beijing, China; Chinese Ancient Medical Book Press. 353 pp.

Peng, Y. & Xiao, P.G. 1993. A review on the resource utilization of Chinese medicinal plants. *Journal of Plant Resources and Environment* 2: (1) 49-55.

Song, Z.J. 1992. Present status of research on Chinese medicines for antiageing. *Chinese Prepared Medicines* 14: (3) 38-40.

Wang, L.S. 1992. Problems in the development of medicinal plant resources. *Chinese Herbal Durgs* 23: (7) 385-387.

Yuan, C.Q., Wang, L.H. & Lu, Y. 1992. The necessity of strengthening the conservation and management of Chinese medicinal plant resources. *Journal of Chinese Traditional Medicines* 17: (1) 3-5.

Zhun Y.L. 1991. Developmental research on Chinese and natural medicines for AIDS. *Journal of Chinese Traditional Medicines*. 16: (12) 707-710.

An Africa-wide overview of medicinal plant harvesting, conservation and health care

A.B. Cunningham
WWF/UNESCO/Kew People and Plants Initiative
P O Box 42
Betty's Bay 7141
South Africa

Abstract

This paper gives an overview of medicinal plant harvesting for the commercial trade in traditional medicines, and its relevance to medicinal plant conservation and the self-sufficiency of traditional medical practitioners. The most vulnerable species are popular, slow reproducing species with specific habitat requirements and a limited distribution. Although in theory sustainable use of bark, roots or whole plants used as herbal medicines is possible, the high level of input of resources in terms of money and manpower required for intensive management of slow-growing species in multiple-species systems is unlikely to be found in most African countries. Cultivation of alternative supply sources of popular, high conservation priority species outside of core conservation areas is therefore essential. Commercial cultivation of high conservation priority species is not a simple solution and at present unlikely to be a profitable exercise for most species due to slow growth rates and low prices paid for traditional medicines. These slow-growing species are a priority for ex-situ conservation and strict protection in core conservation areas. However, the high price paid for some species does make them potential new crop plants for agroforestry systems (e.g. *Warburgia salutaris*, *Garcinia kola*, *G. afzellii*, *G. epunctata* or agricultural production (e.g. *Siphonochilus aethiopicus*) and pilot study commercial production is warranted. The following regions are considered to be priority areas for co-operative action between health care professionals, farmers, horticulturists and conservation biologists: West Africa (Guineo-Congolese region), specifically Ghana, Nigeria and Côte d'Ivoire; East Africa (Kenya, Tanzania, Ethiopia) and south-eastern Africa (Swaziland, South Africa). These are all rapidly urbanizing regions with a high level of endemic plant taxa. The most threatened vegetation types are Afro-montane forest, coastal forests of the Zanzibar-Inhambane regional mosaic and those in the Guineo-Congolese Region.

Introduction

This paper is based on a series of surveys undertaken in Africa during 1986-1989, in order to develop a conservation policy on the herbal medicine trade (Cunningham, 1988a, 1990, 1991, 1993). All of these drew on the local knowledge of traditional medical practitioners (TMPs) and herb traders, and concentrated on commercially sold species in setting priorities for medicinal plant conservation and resource management. From these studies, it was clear that medicinal plant species gathered for commercial purposes represent the most popular and often the most effective (physiologically or psychosomatically) herbal remedies. From historical records it is also clear that the majority of species that were popular in the past are still popular today (e.g.

Erythrophleum lasianthum, *Cassine transvaalensis*, *Alepidea amatymbica* and *Warburgia salutaris* in southern Africa). Commercially sold species thus represent a "short-list" of medicinal plants used nationally, as many species that are used to a limited extent in rural areas are not in demand in urban areas.

In most cases, non-sustainable use of favoured species results from commercial harvesting to supply an urban demand for traditional medicines after clearing due to agricultural or urban associated development had already taken place. The widespread commercial harvesting and sale of the same genera and species throughout their distribution range is also significant (e.g. *Solanum* fruits, *Erythrophleum* bark, *Abrus precatorius* seeds, *Myrothamnus flabellifolius* stems and leaves, and *Swartzia madagascariensis* roots).

Herbal medicine sellers are familiar with the species which are becoming difficult to obtain (because of limited geographical distribution, habitat destruction or over-exploitation). Their insights, coupled with botanical knowledge of the plant species involved, their ecology and distribution, therefore provide an essential source of information for cost-effective surveys (Cunningham, 1991). What is needed is a common methodology applied on the basis of ethnobotanical surveys of markets, as suggested by the IUCN Species Survival Commission Medicinal Plants Specialist Group (MPSG, 1996).

Akerele (1987), Anyinam (1987), Good (1987) and others have pointed out that there is a need, through training and evaluation of effective remedies, to involve TMPs in national health care systems as they are an important and influential group involved in health care. Sustainable use of the major resource base of TMPs - the medicinal plants - is therefore essential.

A hidden economy: dynamics of the commercial trade in medicinal plants

Stimulated by high population growth rates, rapid urbanization, rural unemployment and the value placed on traditional medicines, the national and regional commercial trade in traditional medicines is now greater than at any time in the past. Due to diversity of species used and intertwined religious and socio-economic issues, sustainable use of traditional medicinal plant resources is also the most complex African resource management issue facing conservation agencies, health care professionals and resource users. International export trade also occurs, but is focused on a limited number of species. Constructive resource management and conservation action therefore has to be founded on a clear understanding of the key factors driving medicinal plant use. Where over-exploitation of medicinal plants occurs, it has arisen through three main factors:

Firstly, there has been a decline in the area of distribution of natural vegetation that was, or would have been the source of supply of traditional medicines. An extreme example of this is *Monanthotaxis capea*, which formerly was harvested for its aromatic leaves for a trade from Côte d'Ivoire to Ghana but is now extinct in the wild after the forest reserve in which it occurred was declassified and cleared for agriculture. In addition, supplies of herbal medicines to TMPs are affected by competing uses such as timber logging (e.g. *Pericopsis elata* in Côte d'Ivoire, *Pterocarpus angolensis* in Zambia and Malawi), commercial harvesting for export and extraction of pharmaceuticals, (e.g.

Griffonia simplicifolia and *Prunus africana*), and use for building materials and fuel. A growing demand is thus placed on fewer resources, ultimately threatening those within conservation areas.

Secondly, Africa has the highest rate of urbanization in the world, with urban populations doubling every 14 years as cities grow at 5.1% per annum (Huntley *et al.*, 1989). A large proportion of the urban African population consult traditional practitioners due to the widely held belief that good health, disease, success or misfortune are not chance occurrences, but are due to the action of individuals or ancestral spirits. The urban demand for traditional medicines thus generates a species-specific informal trade network which can extend across international boundaries.

Thirdly, in African countries with large urban populations, medicinal plant use has changed from being a purely specialist activity of traditional medical practitioners to one involving an informal sector group of medicinal plant gatherers. Unlike the rural TMPs who gather medicinal plant material in small quantities, the prime motivation of the commercial gatherers is an economic one. This results in disregard for traditional conservation practices where they exist and an opportunistic scramble for the last bag of bark, bulbs or roots. High rates of unemployment and low levels of formal education (and therefore a low chance of access to the formal job market) have given rise to a flood of popular medicinal plant material to supply the urban demand, keeping prices low and volumes sold high. In the case of medicinal plants harvested and exported for the pharmaceutical industry, prices are also kept low through agreements on prices that do not take resource replacement costs into account.

Urban migration of traditional medical practitioners

A high level of expectations, high unemployment rates, a psychologically stressful environment, and often crowded and unhygienic living conditions are a feature of many urban areas in Africa. Labour migrancy also creates the need to maintain relationships with wives, or find new partners in the urban environment. Under these circumstances, it is therefore not surprising that many of the traditional medicinal plant and animal material sold in urban markets has symbolic or psychosomatic value for luck in finding employment, guarding against jealousy when a person has a job whilst their peer group are unemployed, or love-charms and aphrodisiacs to keep a wife or partner. It is also not surprising that employment options for TMPs increase, as a declining medical : total population ratio is a feature of rapid urbanization. In Lagos, Nigeria, for example, the number of medical doctors increased five-fold since 1955, yet the medical doctor : total population ratio in 1975 was 1:5,000 compared to 1:2,000 in 1955, as provision of western-type medical facilities could not cope with the rapidly growing urban population (Udo, 1987).

Traditional medical practitioners are therefore attracted to urban centres where employment can be rewarding, and studies in Dar es Salaam (Tanzania), Ibadan (Nigeria), Lusaka (Zambia), Kinshasa (Zaire), Kampala (Uganda) and Nairobi (Kenya) have shown that "urban centres are viable and vigorous areas of traditional medicine" (Good & Kimani, 1980). In Zimbabwe this is clearly shown by the higher ratio of TMP : total population in urban areas (1:234) compared to rural areas (1:956) (Gelfand *et al.*, 1985).

This is not always the case, however. In the rural area of Kilungu district, Kenya, rural populations of TMPs averaged 1:224 (herbalists 1:665; traditional birth attendants 1:1640 and diviners also 1:665) while in urban Mathare, the overall ratio was 1:883 (Good, 1987). Rapid urbanization and greater demand for traditional medicines result in an increase in harvesting of medicinal plants from rural areas, a depletion of the rural resource base where certain species are vulnerable to over-exploitation, and consequent problems for primary health care. The same applies to harvesting of medicinal plant material for export and processing into modern pharmaceuticals.

Sustainability and effects of harvesting

It is generally accepted that for any resource, a relationship exists between resources stock, population size and sustainable rate of harvest. Low stocks are likely to produce small sustainable yields, particularly if the target species is slow-growing and slow-reproducing. Conversely, large stocks of species with a high biomass production and short time to reproductive maturity could be expected to produce high sustainable yields, particularly if competitive interaction is reduced by "thinning". There is also a clear relationship between the part of the plant harvested, harvesting method used, and the impact of these on the plant.

Traditional medicinal plants

Demand for fast-growing species with a wide distribution, high natural population density and high percentage seed set is easily met, particularly where leaves, seeds, flowers or fruits are used. The common sale and use of medicinal plant leaves as a source of medicine in Côte d'Ivoire (and possibly other parts of West Africa) is therefore highly significant as it differs markedly from the high frequency of roots, bark or bulbs at markets in the Southern African region. Throughout Malawi, Mozambique, Zambia, Zimbabwe, Lesotho, Swaziland and particularly South Africa, herbal material that is dried (roots, bark) or has a long shelf-life (bulbs, seeds, fruits) dominates herbal medicine markets. In comparison, six sellers in Abidjan, Côte d'Ivoire, primarily sold leaf material (20-41 species), followed by roots (1 16 species), bark (0-8 species) and whole plants (0-3 species) a situation that was typical of the 111 traditional medicine sellers. The exception in Côte d'Ivoire are sellers bringing material from Burkina Faso and Mali, who sell more root and bark material. The situation with chewing stick sellers in Côte d'Ivoire and other parts of West Africa is somewhat different however, as stems and roots are the major plant parts used, with consequent higher impact on favoured species.

Despite limited information on population biology of medicinal plants, it is possible to group target plant species according to demand, plant life-form, part used, distribution and abundance (Cunningham, 1988a, 1991). Of little concern to TMPs or conservation biologists are the large category of traditional medicinal plants where there is no threat at all, and demand easily meets supply due to (a) unpopularity of the species; (b) low human population densities and low demand in relation to wild stocks; (c) lack of development of a commercial trade to urban areas, in which case only a selective harvesting is done by TMPs and not by commercial gatherers; and (d) a situation where demand is high, and commercial harvesting takes place, but supplies meet demand as the species concerned are abundant, widely distributed and the impact of harvesting is low (due to the resilience of the plant source, rapid growth and reproductive rates or the use of leaves, seeds or fruits rather than bark, roots, bulbs or the whole plant).

From a conservation viewpoint on an Africa-wide scale, there are two categories of medicinal plants that are of concern. Firstly, where slow growing species with a limited distribution are the focus of commercial gathering with demand exceeding supply. The consequent expansion of gathering to further and further afield (as incentives to collect are covered by rising prices for the target species) results in the species being endangered regionally, with widespread depletion of rural resource bases of TMPs (e.g. *Warburgia salutaris* in East and southern Africa; *Siphonochilus aethiopicus* in Swaziland and South Africa). Endemic species with a very localized distribution are a particular problem. Southern African examples of this are *Ledebouria hypoxidoides*, an endemic of the eastern Cape region, South Africa, where herbalists were observed removing the last bulbs from the type locality near Grahamstown (F. Venter, pers. comm.) and *Mystacidium millari*, also a South African endemic which is threatened due to harvesting and commercial sale as a traditional medicine in the nearby city of Durban, South Africa (Cunningham, 1988a). Secondly, where a species may be popular, but not endangered due to its widespread distribution, but where habitat change through commercial harvesting is cause for concern. *Trichilia emetica* and *Albizia adianthifolia* for example, are not a high species conservation priority in southern Africa, although they are a popular source of traditional medicines. However, ring-barking in "conserved" forests and consequent development of canopy gaps (which change forest structure and can lead to influx of invasive exotic species) is of concern in forest habitat conservation.

Both problems affect protected area management, as core conservation areas will ultimately become the focus of harvesting efforts for favoured species if they are no longer available elsewhere.

Quantities in local or national trade

Information on the quantities of plant material being harvested or sold (whether for the local trade as traditional medicines, or for export and extraction of active ingredients) is sparse. Apart from placing the quantities required from cultivation into perspective, it is also of little relevance unless expressed in terms of impact of the species concerned. In South Africa, harvesting from wild populations of certain species is on a scale that is cause for concern amongst conservation organizations and rural herbalists, and a listing of priority species is available (Cunningham, 1988a). The same concern also applies to some chewing stick sources (e.g. *Garcinia afzelii* in West Africa. The only quantitative data on volume of plant material sold locally is from South Africa (Cunningham, 1990, 1993; Osborne *et al.*, 1994; Williams, 1996). The scale of this trade is such that it can have an immense impact on wild populations. *Stangeria eriopus* cycads collected from the wild, for example, which are sold at a rate of over 3,000 per month, are also sold in the city of Durban, South Africa as an *intelezi* (protective charm), posing a conservation problem which Osborne *et al.* (1994) have termed "an enigma of the South African situation to which it is difficult to find a solution".

Table 1. African medicinal plant species in international trade showing quantities traded, exporting and importing countries. Percentage of total demand are given where posssible.

Family species	Part used	Export country	Year	Quantity traded in tons/yr	Import country and % of demand imported	Source of collection *	Reference**
Annonaceae							
Dennettia tripetala	?	Ghana				w	1
Apocynaceae							
Hunteria eburnea	bark	Ghana				w	1
Rauvolfia vomitoria	root	Zaire Rwanda Mozambique				c	
Strophanthus gratus	fruit	Cameroon	1985-86 1990-91	1.1	Luxembourg Belgium (38%)	w	8
Strophanthus kombe	fruit				Italy (23%) Holland (13%) Germany (12%) France (11%) Spain (2.4%)	w	3
Tabernaemontana elegans	seed	Mozambique	1981	0.6		w	9
Voacanga africana	seed	Cameroon Côte d'Ivoire	1985-86 1990-91		France	w, c	3
Voacanga thouarsii	seed	Cameroon				w, c	1, 2, 5
Combretaceae							
Terminalia sericea	bark	Mozambique		24-25	Germany ?	w	9
Euphorbiaceae							
Ricinus communis	seed	Mozambique	1982	50		n	9
Fabaceae							
Duparquetia orchidacea		Ghana				w	1
Griffonia simplicifolia	seed	Ghana Côte d'Ivoire, Cameroon		75-80	Germany	w	1, 2, 5
Physostigma venenosum	fruit	Côte d'Ivoire, Nigeria				w	1, 2

Liliaceae							
Gloriosa superba	seed	Mozambique	1981	0.1			9
Menispermaceae							
Jateorhiza palmata	root	Tanzania				w	4
	root	Mozambique		0.7-24			9
Pedaliaceae							
Harpagophytum procumbens	root	Namibia Mozambique Botswana	 1981	200 9	Germany (80.4%) France (12.8%) Italy (1.5%) USA (1.0%) South Africa (1.2%)	w	4, 9
Harpagophytum zeyheri	root	Namibia Mozambique Botswana				w	4
Ochnaceae							
Brackenridgea zanguebarica	bark	Mozambique	1981	0.1		w	9
Rosaceae							
Prunus africana	bark	Cameroon Madagascar Kenya, Zaire Uganda	1995	3190	France Italy Spain	w	3, 6
Rubiaceae							
Corynanthe pachyceras	?	Ghana				w	1
Pausinystalia johimbe	bark	Cameroon	1985-91	286	Holland (65%) Germany (18.3%) Belgium/Luxembourg (10.9%) France (5.9%)	w	3, 5, 8

*Source of collection: w = wild; c = cultivated; n = naturalised

**References: 1. Abbiw (1990); 2. Ake Assi (pers. comm.); 3. Cunningham & Mbenkum (1993); 4. Nott (1986); 5. J. Seyani (pers. comm.); 6. FAO (1986); 7. Catalano *et al.* (1985); 8. Seme (1989); 9. Atal (1993).

Quantities in international trade

An average of 25% of prescription drugs sold in the USA during the period 1959 - 1973 contained active principles still derived from higher plants (Farnsworth & Soejarto, 1985) significantly overlapping with plant sources used in traditional medicine. Farnsworth (1988) for example, points out that of the 119 chemicals derived from higher plants which are used for modern pharmaceuticals on a global scale, 74% have similar or related uses in traditional medicine. Like the trade in traditional medicines to cities however, neither the impact of harvesting nor the cost of replacing these resources seems to have been taken into account. For this reason, even when the technology for chemical synthesis is available, it can be cheaper for pharmaceutical companies to extract the active ingredients. In the mid-1970s, for example, the cost of producing reserpine by chemical synthesis was $1.25 per g, compared to $0.75 per g by commercial extraction from *Rauvolfia vomitoria* roots (Oldfield, 1984). If replacement costs and sustainable use were taken into consideration, this may not be the case.

While data on the quantities of raw material harvested for export are limited, even less data are available on the environmental impact of harvesting. From what little evidence is available, it is clear, however, that large quantities of material are collected from the wild (Table 1) and that harvesting can be very destructive (Cunningham and Mbenkum, 1993). For example, Ake-Assi (pers. comm.) reports that although only fruits are required, commercial gatherers in Côte d'Ivoire chop down *Griffonia simplicifolia* vines and *Voacanga africana* and *V. thouarsii* trees in order to obtain the fruits. Concern has been expressed about a similar situation in Indonesia (Rifai and Kartawinata, 1991).

Sustainability and the impact of commercial harvesting

Due to the number of species involved and the limited amount of information available on biomass, primary production and demography of indigenous medicinal plants, no detailed assessment is possible of sustainable off-take from natural populations. Even if these data were available, their value would be questionable due to the intensive management inputs required for managing sustainable use of vulnerable species in cases where demand exceeds supply. What can be done is to identify the categories of medicinal plant species that are most vulnerable to over-exploitation by combining the insights of herbal medicine sellers with our knowledge of plant biology and distribution (Cunningham, 1990).

The most vulnerable species are the popular, slow-growing, slow-reproducing species with specific habitat requirements and a limited distribution. Although in theory sustainable use of bark, roots or whole plants used as herbal medicines is possible, the high levels of money and manpower required for intensive management of slow-growing species in multiple-species systems are unlikely to be found in most African countries. Cultivation of alternative supply sources of popular, high conservation priority species outside of core conservation areas is therefore essential. However, commercial cultivation of high conservation priority species is not a simple solution and, at present, unlikely to be a profitable exercise for most species due to their slow growth rates and the low prices paid for traditional medicines. These slow-growing species are a priority for *ex-situ* conservation and strict protection in core conservation areas. However, the high price paid for some species does make them potential new crop plants for agroforestry systems (e.g.

Warburgia salutaris), *Garcinia kola*, *G. afzelii*, *G. epunctata*) or agricultural production (e.g. *Siphonochilus aethiopicus*), and pilot study commercial production is warranted. Priority regions for co-operative action between health care professionals are considered to be the rapidly urbanizing areas with a high level of endemic taxa, particularly West Africa (Guineo-Congolese region), specifically Ghana, Nigeria and Côte d'Ivoire; East Africa (Kenya, Tanzania, Ethiopia) and south-eastern Africa (Swaziland, South Africa). Most threatened vegetation types are Afro-montane forest, coastal forests of the Zanzibar-Inhambane regional mosaic and those in the Guineo-Congolese region.

Commercial gatherers of medicinal plant material, whether for national or international trade, are poor people whose main aim is earning money, and not resource management. Unsustainably high levels of exploitation are not a new problem, although the problem has escalated in regions with large urban areas and high levels of urbanization since the 1960s. Prior to 1898, local extermination of *Mondia whitei* had been recorded in the Durban area of South Africa due to collection of its roots for commercial sale. By 1900, *Siphonochilus natalensis* (now considered synonymous with *Siphonochilus aethiopicus*) had disappeared from its only known localities in the Inanda and Umhloti valleys due to a trade to Lesotho (Medley-Wood & Franks, 1911). This occurred despite a traditional seasonal restriction on harvesting this species. By 1938, all that could be found of *Warburgia salutaris* in Natal and Zululand was "poor coppices, every year cut right down to the bottom" (Gerstner, 1938). With these few exceptions, most botanical and forestry records reflect the impact of commercial collection of *Ocotea bullata* bark due to the importance of this species for timber (see Cunningham, 1993). The situation would appear to be similar in Kenya, where Kokwaro (1991) records that some of the largest *Warburgia salutaris* and *Olea capensis* subsp. *welwitschii* trees have been completely ring-barked and have died as a result. Heavy commercial exploitation of *Prunus africana* trees has devastated populations in Cameroon (Cunningham & Mbenkum, 1993) and Madagascar (Walter and Rakotonirina, 1995). In Zimbabwe, due to the high demand and limited distribution of this species, the situation is worse, and all that remains of *Warburgia salutaris* wild populations are a few coppice shoots. In Côte d'Ivoire, *Garcinia afzelii* is considered threatened due to harvesting for the chewing stick trade (Ake-Assi, 1988). Destructive harvesting of *Griffonia simplicifolia*, *Voacanga thuoarsii* and *V.africana* fruits (for the international pharmaceutical market) through felling of the plants bearing them is also of concern. In Sapoba Forest Reserve, Nigeria, despite traditional restrictions on bark removal, Hardie (1963) observed how the trunk of a large *Okoubaka aubrevillei* tree (a very rare species in West Africa) "was much scarred where pieces of bark had been removed". There appears to be nothing published on the current status of this species. Botanical records are scanty, particularly for bulbous or herbaceous species, where little remains to indicate former occurrence after the plant has been removed. It would therefore be useful to carry out damage assessments for exported species such as *Okoubaka aubrevillei*, *Garcinia afzelii* and *G. kola* in West Africa (Ghana, Côte d'Ivoire, Nigeria) and *Warburgia salutaris* in Kenya, Tanzania and Zimbabwe, and assessments of the impact of *Pausinystalia johimbe* bark harvesting in Cameroon and *Griffonia simplicifolia* in Ghana.

Field observation has shown a high level of damage to *Prunus africana* populations in north and west Cameroon (Cunningham and Mbenkum, 1993). In South Africa, bark damage assessments using a 7-point scale (Cunningham, 1990) were carried out for key "indicator species" (medicinal plants chosen for their relatively slow growth rate). Information was also recorded on popularity as a source of traditional medicines, scarcity. Bark damage assessments confirmed most of the observations of herbalists and herb traders (Cunningham, 1988a, 1990), the exceptions being species that were scarce not because of over-exploitation, but due to limited geographical distribution in the region, such as *Acacia xanthoploea* and *Synaptolepsis kirkii*. They also demonstrate the very different situation to customary subsistence use, and this fact needs to be taken into account in legislation covering protected area management where conservation of biotic diversity is a primary objective. Although the degree of bark damage varies, the level of damage at all sites where commercial gathering takes place is high and involves mainly trees in the larger diameter size classes. What is significant is that extensive damage has taken place in State Forest, which is theoretically set aside for maintenance of habitat and species diversity (Cunningham, 1988a, 1990). In the Malowe State Forest, Transkei, South Africa, if coppice stems of less than 2cm diameter are excluded, then the level of damage to *Curtisia dentata* and *Ocotea bullata* trees encountered amounted to 51% and 57% of trees with more than half the trunk bark removed. All *Warburgia salutaris* trees found outside strict conservation areas in Natal were ring-barked, and many of those inside conserved areas had their bark removed as well.

Even fewer data are available on the impact of harvesting bulbs, roots, or whole plants although local depletion of *Stangeria eriopsius*, *Gnidia kraussiana* and *Alepidea amatymbica* is known from Natal, South Africa. There has also been a marked reduction in the number of the Afro-montane forest climber *Dumasia villosa*, which is sold in large quantities in herbal medicine shops (Cunningham, 1988a). In northern Namibia, *Protea gauguedi* populations have become locally extinct despite attempts at protection by the conservation department. It is worth noting that this has taken place in response to demands placed by a local trade in an area where urban centres are small. Commercial harvesting of *Harpagophytum procumbens* tubers in Botswana removed up to 66% of plants (Leloup, 1984). In Namibia, however, this species was not considered threatened as the 200 tons exported per annum only represented 2% of the total stocks (de Bruine *et al.* (1977) as cited by Nott, 1986).

Increasing scarcity of popular species is accompanied by an increasing prices, which in turn provide greater incentives to harvest remaining stocks. The effects of this are firstly, decreased self-sufficiency of traditional medical practitioners as local sources of favoured species decline, and secondly, higher prices which people have to pay for those species. As demand is one of the root causes of over-exploitation, the most popular and effective species are most vulnerable.

Conservation through cultivation as an alternative

Provision of an alternative to over-exploitation of traditional medicinal plants through cultivation was suggested over 50 years ago in South Africa for scarce and effective species such as *Alepidea amatymbica* (Gerstner, 1938) and *Warburgia salutaris* (Gerstner, 1946). Until six years ago, no large scale cultivation had taken place. There are two main reasons for this, and both are applicable elsewhere in Africa: (i) a lack of institutional support for production and dissemination of key species for cultivation; and (ii) the low prices paid for traditional medicinal plants by herbal medicine traders and urban herbalists.

If cultivation is to succeed in providing an alternative supply source to improve self-sufficiency of TMPs and take harvesting pressure off wild stocks, then plants have to be produced cheaply and in large quantity. Any cultivation for meeting the urban demand will be competing with material harvested from the wild that is supplied onto the market by commercial gatherers, who have incurred no input costs for cultivation. Prices therefore increase with scarcity as the transport costs and search time increase for the long-distance trade. At present, low prices (whether for local or international pharmaceutical trade) ensure that few species can be marketed at a high enough price to make cultivation profitable. Even fewer of these are in the category most threatened by over-exploitation.

In all cases where cultivation has taken place, whether in Europe, Asia or Africa, the crops chosen are those yielding good economic returns or a high level of resource returns (e.g. multiple use species for fruits, shade and medicinal properties). These are either fast growing species, or plants where a sustainable harvest is possible (e.g. resins (*Boswellia*), leaves (*Catha edulis*)).

With few exceptions, prices paid to gatherers are very low, bearing no relation to annual sustainable off-take. In many cases, they are collected from open access, rather than limited access or privately owned sites. To make a living, commercial medicinal plant gatherers therefore "mine" rather than manage these resources. If cultivation of tree species is to be a viable proposition or an income-generating activity, the flood of cheap bark/roots "mined" from wild stocks should be reduced through better protection of conserved forests in order to bring prices to a realistic level. Alternatively, wild populations will have to decline further before cultivation becomes a viable option.

Cultivation for profit is therefore restricted to a small number of high-priced and/or fast-growing species such as *Warburgia salutaris*, *Alepidea amatymbica*, *Cassia abbreviata*, *Haworthia limifolia* and *Siphonochilus aethiopicus* in southern Africa and *Garcinia afzelii* and *Monanthotaxis capea* in West Africa.

Although a few of these species are threatened in the wild (e.g. *Garcinia afzelii* and *Warburgia salutaris*), low prices ensure that few slow-growing species are cultivated. With the declining economic state of many African countries, it is unlikely that subsidized production of these species will occur, and collection of seed or cuttings for establishment of field gene banks (for recalcitrant fruiting species) and seed banks must therefore be seen as an urgent priority.

Strong support and commitment are necessary if cultivation is to succeed as a means of meeting the requirements of processing plants for pharmaceuticals (whether for local consumption or export) or urban demand for chewing sticks and traditional medicinal plants. If cultivation does not take place on a large enough scale to meet demand, it merely becomes a convenient bit of "window dressing" masking the continued exploitation of wild populations. The regional demand for *Scilla natalensis* in Natal, South Africa is 300,000 bulbs/year, which are at least 8-10 year old from the wild. On a 6-year rotation under cultivation at the same planting densities as those used by Gentry *et al.* (1987) for *Urginea maritima*, 70 ha would be required (Cunningham, 1988a). Due to their slow growth rates, the rotational area required for tree species would be far greater, the total area being dependent on demand.

The success of cultivation also depends on the attitude of TMPs to cultivated material, and this varies from place to place. In Botswana, TMPs said that cultivated material was unacceptable, as cultivated plants did not have the power of material collected from the wild. Discussions with some 400 TMPs in South Africa over a two-year period showed general acceptance of cultivated material as an alternative. Similarly, TMPs in the Malolotja area, Swaziland accepted cultivation as a viable alternative. In both countries there is a tradition of growing succulent plant species near homesteads to ward off lightning. Similarly, in Ghana, West Africa, plants of spiritual significance such as *Datura metel*, *Pergularia daemia*, *Leptadenia hastata* and *Scoparia dulcis* are tended around villages. Therefore, although little is known about attitudes to cultivation of medicinal plants in West Africa, it is possible that TMPs would be in favour of cultivation of alternative supply sources.

A good model to follow may be the Thailand example where (i) a project for cultivation of medicinal plants of known efficacy has been initiated in about 1,000 villages (ii) traditional household remedies, with improved formulae, are produced as compressed tablets packed in foil and distributed to "drug co-operatives" set up through a Drug and Medical Project Fund in more than 45,000 villages as well as in community hospitals (Desawadi, 1988). Wondergem *et al.* (1989) have already drawn from the Thailand experience in making recommendations regarding primary health care in Ghana.

References

Abbiw, D.K. 1990. *Useful Plants of Ghana*. Kew, UK; Royal Botanic Gardens. 337 pp.

Ake-Assi, L. 1988. Plantes médicinales: Quelques légumineuses utilisées dans la médecine de tradition africaine en Côte d'Ivoire. *Monographs in Systematic Botany from the Missouri Botanical Gardens* 25: 309-313.

Akerele, O. 1987. The best of both worlds: bringing traditional medicine up to date. *Soc. Sci. Med.* 24: 177-181.

Anyinam, C. 1987. Availability, accessibility, acceptability and adaptability: four attributes of African ethnomedicine. *Social Science and Medicine* 25: 803-811.

Catalano, S., Ferretti, M., Marsili, A. & Morelli, I. 1984. New constituents of *Prunus africana* bark extract. *Journal of Natural Products* 47: 910.

Cunningham, A.B. 1988a. *An Investigation of the Herbal Medicine Trade in Natal/KwaZulu*. Investigational Report No.29, Institute of Natural Resources, University of Natal, Pietermaritzburg, South Africa.

Cunningham, A.B. 1988b. Collection of wild plant foods in Tembe Thonga society: a guide to Iron Age gathering activities? *Annals of the Natal Museum* 29: (2) 433-446.

Cunningham, A.B. 1990. Man and medicines: the exploitation and conservation of traditional Zulu medicinal plants. *Mitteilungen aus dem Institut für allgemeine Botanik, Hamburg*. 23: 979-990. Proceedings of the 1988 AETFAT Congress, Hamburg.

Cunningham, A.B. 1991. Development of a conservation policy on commercially exploited medicinal plants : A case study from southern Africa. In : Heywood, V., Synge, H & Akerele, O (eds). *Conservation of Medicinal Plants*. Cambridge, UK; Cambridge University Press. pp. 337-358.

Cunningham, A.B. 1993. *African Medicinal Plants: Setting Priorities at the Interface between Conservation and Primary Health Care*. Working Paper 1, WWF/UNESCO/Kew People and Plants Initiative. Paris, France; UNESCO.

Cunningham, A.B. & Mbenkum, F.T. 1993. *Sustainability of harvesting Prunus africana bark in Cameroon: a medicinal plant in international trade*. Working Paper 2, pp. 1-28, WWF/UNESCO/Kew People and Plants Initiative. Paris, France; UNESCO.

Desawadi, P. 1988. The conservation of medicinal plants used in primary health care in Thailand. Paper given at the *International Consultation on Conservation of Medicinal Plants, 21-27 March, 1988, Chiang Mai, Thailand.*

Farnsworth, N.R. 1988. Screening plants for new medicines. In: Wilson, E.O. (Ed) *Biodiversity*. Washington, D.C., USA; National Academy Press. pp 83-97.

Farnsworth, N.R. & Soejarto, D.D. 1985. Potential consequence of plant extinction in the United States on the current and future availability of prescription drugs. *Economic Botany* 39: 231-240.

Gelfand, M., Mavi, Drummond, R.B. & Ndemera, B. 1985. *The Traditional Medical Practitioner in Zimbabwe*. Harare, Zimbabwe; Mambo Press.

Gentry, H.S., Verbiscar, A.J. & Branigan, T.F. 1987. Red Squill (*Urginea maritima,* Liliaceae). *Economic Botany* 41: (2) 267-282.

Gerstner, J. 1938. A preliminary checklist of Zulu names of plants. *Bantu Studies* 12: 215-236.

Gerstner, J. 1939. A preliminary checklist of Zulu names of plants. *Bantu Studies* 13: 307-326.

Gerstner, J. 1946. Some factors affecting the perpetuation of our indigenous flora. *Journal of South African Forestry Association* 13: 4-11.

Good, C.M. 1987. *Ethnomedical Systems in Africa: Patterns of Traditional Medicine in Rural and Urban Kenya*. The Guildford Press, Kenya.

Good, C.M. & Kimani, V.N. 1980. Urban traditional medicine: A Nairobi case study. *East African Medical Journal* 57: 301-316.

Hardie, A.D.K. 1963. Okoubaka - a rare juju tree. *Nigerian Field* 27: (2) 70-72.

Huntley, B.R., Siegfried & Sunter, C. 1989. *South African Environments into the 21st Century*. Cape Town, South Africa; Human and Rousseau.

Kokwaro, J.O. 1991. Conservation of medicinal plants in Kenya. In: Heywood, V., Synge, H & Akerele, O (eds). Conservation of Medicinal Plants. Cambridge, UK; Cambridge University Press. pp.315-320.

Leloup, S. 1984. The grapple plant project: an ecophysiological approach of the influence of harvest on the population dynamics of the Grapple plant *Harpagophytum procumbens* DC. National Institute for Development Research and Documentation.

MPSG. 1996. Towards the "Top 50" medicinal plants. *Medicinal Plants Specilaist Group Newsletter* No. 2. SSC, IUCN. Gland, Switzerland; World Conservation Union.

Medley-Wood, J. & Franks, M. 1911. *Kaempferia natalensis* Scltr. & Schum. *The Naturalist* (Natal Science Society) 1: 112-115.

Nott, K. 1986. A survey of the harvesting and export of *Harpagophytum procumbens* and *Harpagophytum zeyheri* in SWA/Namibia. Unpublished Report, Etosha Ecological Institute,Okaukuejo, Namibia.

Oldfield, M. 1984. *The Value of Conserving Genetic Resources*. Washington, D.C., USA; US Department of Interior.

Osborne, R., Grove, A., Oh, P., Mabry, T.J., Ng, J.C. & Seawright, A.A. 1994. The magical and medicinal usage of *Stangeria eriopus* in South Africa. *Journal of Ethnopharmacology* 43: (2) 67-72.

Seme, P.M. 1989. *Situation de l'Exploitation des Plantes Médicinales au Cameroun*. Centre Universitaire de Dschang, Ministère de l'Enseignement Supérieur, de l"Informatique et de la Recherche Scientifique, Cameroun.

Udo, K. 1987. *A Human Geography of Africa*. London, UK; Longmans..

Walter , S. & Rakotonirina, J-C. R. 1995. *L'exploitation de Prunus africanum à Madagascar*. PCDI Zahamena et la Direction des Eaux et Forêts, Antananarivo, Madagascar.

White, F. 1983. *The Vegetation of Africa*. Paris, France; UNESCO. 356 pp.

Williams, V L. 1996. The Witwatersrand multi trade. *Veld and Flora* 82: 12-14.

Wondergem, P., Senah, K.A. & Glover, E.K. 1989. *Herbal Drugs in Primary Health Care*. Amsterdam, Netherlands; Royal Tropical Institute.

Biodiversity conservation and the application of Amazonian medicinal plants in the control of malaria

William Milliken
Royal Botanic Gardens, Kew
Richmond, Surrey, TW9 3AE, UK
Tel: 0181 332 5783/ Fax:0181 332 5278 / Email: W.Milliken@rbgkew.org.uk

Valuing the rainforest

The potential monetary value of rainforests, and its implications for the conservation of biodiversity, have now been discussed at length by a number of authors, some of whom have attempted to quantify this value (e.g. Peters, Gentry and Mendelsohn, 1989). These discussions were spawned by the rationale that there must be means of rainforest exploitation which are more financially viable than their conversion to short-term agricultural land or cattle pasture. This in turn responds to the assumption that unless a financially viable conservation option is presented to the developing countries in which most rainforests are found, then they will eventually be destroyed for short-term gain. The potential income generated by sustainable logging, extractivism (non-timber forest products), ecotourism and biodiversity prospecting have all been considered in this context. Of these, it is biodiversity prospecting, or more specifically the search for new pharmaceutical products, which has tended to generate the most enthusiasm and rhetoric. No rainforest conservation campaign leaflet is complete without a mention of the countless species with un-investigated pharmacological properties which are disappearing every day. On paper, at least, the proceeds of biodiversity prospecting also appear to present the highest potential financial returns from the rainforest. In spite of the relatively low 'hit rates' obtained by random pharmacological screening, the diversity of currently un-investigated species within even a small tract of rainforest, combined with the enormous profits which can eventually be generated by a successful 'hit', suggest that substantial capital values can be attached to them. Furthermore, agreements such as the Costa Rican INBIO/Merck contract indicate that in certain circumstances there might indeed be viable means of turning this potential value to good advantage for conservation.

Anti-malarial plants of Roraima

Between 1993 and 1995 a survey of the plant species used in the treatment of malaria was conducted in Roraima, the northernmost State of Brazil. Data were collected from seven indigenous groups in the region (the Yanomami, Macuxi, Maiongong, Wapixana, Taurepang, Ingaricó and Wai-Wai), and also from representatives of the non-indigenous populations. At least 99 plant species, of 82 genera and 41 families, were found to be used specifically in the treatment of malaria. Of these, only 22 appear to have been reported previously in the literature as being used to treat malaria elsewhere. Fifty-three of these species occur in *terra firme* or riverside forest, 17 in natural savanna vegetation, 20 in secondary vegetation or waste ground, and 18 are cultivated. The plants were taxonomically diverse: of the 41 families only eight were represented by more than 3 species. These were the Leguminosae, Rubiaceae, Apocynaceae, Compositae, Euphorbiaceae, Myrtaceae, Piperaceae and Solanaceae. Further details of these plants are to be published elsewhere (Milliken, 1996a, 1996bb). In these publications, in an effort to protect the intellectual property rights of the people who furnished the information, the plants have only been identified to the level of species in cases where the use of that plant as a malaria remedy has already been published, or where its properties are so widely known that its use could not realistically be said to be the intellectual property of any particular group of people.

The logical means of identifying novel anti-malarial compounds is to follow the leads from traditional medicine, and yet the greater part of the (comparatively little) research carried out in this field has to a large extent been based on randomly selected species. There is a very strong case for following up these ethnobotanical leads (Balick 1994, Cox 1994), which is supported by the results of the relatively few anti-malarial studies which have done so (e.g. Phillipson *et al.*, 1987; Phillipson & Wright, 1991a; 1991b; Brandão, Botelho & Krettli, 1985; Brandão *et al.*, 1992). At present, the results of the screening of the plants collected in Roraima are still at a preliminary stage, and do not merit analysis. However, the initial results indicate a far higher percentage incidence of anti-malarial activity *in vitro* than, for example, those of the massive random screening carried out by Spencer *et al.* (1947).

The number of species used in the treatment of this one disease, solely within a relatively small part of the Amazon, is on the face of it remarkable. It emphasizes not only how little we (the outsiders) still know about the medicinal properties of Amazonian plant species, and of the true scope of existing indigenous knowledge of those properties, but also of the enormous potential which still genuinely seems to exist for the discovery of new and viable remedies for major diseases among those plants. In the case of malaria, there is an urgent global need for such new and effective medicines, as resistance to 'traditional' quinine-based compounds continues to develop in the most serious form of the disease, cerebral malaria (*Plasmodium falciparum*), at an alarming rate.

However exciting the implications of the results of this research may be, at present the search for new anti-malarials and its potential rewards do not immediately appear to be a particularly good advertisement for the conservation benefits of biodiversity prospecting. Malaria, being a disease primarily restricted to the poorer countries of the world, cannot compete with the diseases which preoccupy the developed world in terms of being a potential pharmaceutical gold-mine. As a consequence, the amount of commercial-sector research being conducted in this field is minimal. However, if the climatic changes which are predicted as a result of global warming actually take place, this situation could change significantly. Martin and Lefebvre (1995) estimate that this process could increase the range of malaria by up to 28%, by expanding the area in which the ambient temperature and climatic conditions are suitable - at least for part of the year - for its transmission. The areas where malaria transmission is seasonal, and thus most likely to provoke severe epidemics on account of the lower resistance in local populations, may increase by as much as 55%.

Unless one subscribes to the belief that the medicinal properties of plants are the result of divine providence, there is no reason to believe that remedies for diseases which are *not* endemic to rainforest regions should be any less abundant among their plants than remedies for those which are. There really may be cures for AIDS, cancer, asthma and heart disease amongst them. The capacities of the people of these regions or countries to investigate and exploit this potential is, in many cases, limited by a lack of resources and expertise. As a result, if anybody is likely to exploit and profit from the biodiversity of the rainforest, it will be the multi-national pharmaceutical giants. The percentage return to the country of origin, if any, will depend upon the care with which an agreement has been worked out in advance, and on the level of honesty and selflessness of the people involved. Whatever happens, the percentage will inevitably be low. Will this small return be judged by those countries to have justified the 'investment' which it has made in the conservation of rainforest for biodiversity prospecting?

This discussion is missing one crucial point, and one which tends to be missed or dismissed with frightening frequency by developers, national authorities and conservationists alike. The point is that we are discussing rainforests as if they were nothing more than a series of spectacular biodiversity reservoirs, and ignoring the fact that in general they are somebody else's lands over which we (including the national authorities of the countries in which the rainforests occur) do not have the right to make decisions. The resources belong to the indigenous peoples who inhabit these forests, and who rely upon them for their livelihoods.

Anti-malarial plants and conservation

The potential for influencing biodiversity conservation, if there is one, played no part in the conception of this project nor in its execution. What, though, might be the role of research into these northern Amazonian anti-malarials in the promotion of biodiversity conservation? Almost certainly not as a means of identifying a source of funds sufficiently great to guarantee preservation of the rainforests of the region. This has already been discussed. But as a means of helping to support the indigenous peoples who inhabit those forests, and thereby supporting the most careful and effective custodians of their biodiversity? Perhaps. If a commercial anti-malarial product were to be developed from one of the plants collected during this survey, then the percentage of the profits which would theoretically (and rightfully) return to the people who provided the information could potentially bring them significant benefits. At present the greatest need of many of these peoples is for guaranteed rights to their traditional lands, and a source of income could conceivably help them to secure these rights.

One uncomfortable but nonetheless valid consideration is the potentially negative effect which a more effective system of malaria control, whether through the application of new plant products or the use of local plants themselves, might have on the conservation of biodiversity. Malaria, which generally speaking coincides in its geographical range with the areas of greatest global biodiversity, is estimated by the World Health Organization to cause between one and two million deaths per year (principally in Africa). Effective control of the disease would inevitably place a greater population pressure on the natural resources in these areas.

In fact, this project was not aimed at finding new anti-malarial products for world-wide use, but at identifying the most effective locally available medicines for local use. Malaria arrived relatively recently among many of the indigenous communities of Roraima, on the heels of the disastrous gold-rush which swept through the region at the end of the 1980s and the beginning of the 1990s. Lack of previous experience of malaria on an epidemic scale left the more isolated of these communities, such as the Yanomami, in a very precarious situation, some of them having little or no knowledge of how to treat it with locally available resources. Many people died. Suitable resources evidently do appear to exist, however, as demonstrated by the results of this survey, and it is hoped that by identifying the most effective regional anti-malarial plants, and by disseminating information on how they are used, it will be possible to diminish the dependence which some of these indigenous communities have developed on external medical support.

Theoretically, any development which supports the autonomy of indigenous people should strengthen their ability to remain as custodians of their own territories, thereby (incidentally) assisting in the conservation of biodiversity. It would be naive and unrealistic, however, to imagine that such developments are of any great consequence in the face of the greater issues which govern whether or not indigenous peoples are to be able to retain their traditional ways of life and their lands. Northern Amazonian Brazil is a prime example of this conflict of interests. One could promote and encourage the use of locally available medicines and the sustainable use of forest resources until blue in the face, but in truth all of this is fairly irrelevant when viewed in the context of gold-mining, ranching, logging and the lack of sincerety among local and national politicians who support these activities on the lands of indigenous peoples and who consistently and deliberately fail to recognize their rights.

References

Balick, M.J. 1994. Ethnobotany, drug development and biodiversity conservation - exploring the linkages. In: Prance, G.T., Chadwick, D.J. & Marsh, J. (eds) *Ethnobotany and the Search for New Drugs*. Ciba Foundation Symposium 185. New York, USA; John Wiley & Sons. pp. 4-24.

Brandão, M.G.L., Botelho, M.G.A. & Krettli, A.U. 1985. Quimoterapia experimental antimalárica com produtos naturais: uma abordagem mais racional?. *Ciência e Cultura* 37: (7) 1152-1163.

Brandão, M.G.L., Grandi, T.S.M., Rocha, E.M.M., Sawyer, D.R. & Krettli, A.U. 1992. Survey of medicinal plants used as antimalarials in the Amazon. *Journal of Ethnopharmacology* 36: 175-182.

Cox, P.A. 1994. The ethnobotanical approach to drug discovery: strengths and limitations. In: Prance, G.T., Chadwick, D.J. & Marsh, J. (eds) *Ethnobotany and the Search for New Drugs*. Ciba Foundation Symposium 185. New York, USA; John Wiley & Sons. pp. 25-41.

Martin, P.H. & Lefebvre, M.G. 1995. Malaria and climate: sensitivity of malaria potential transmission to climate. *Ambio* 24: (4) 200-207.

Milliken, W. 1996a. Malaria and anti-malarial plants in Roraima, Brazil. *Tropical Doctor* (in press).

Milliken, W. 1996b. Traditional anti-malarial medicine in Roraima, Brazil. Economic Botany (in press).

Peters, C.M., Gentry, A.H. & Mendelsohn, R.O. 1989. Valuation of an Amazonian forest. *Nature* 339: 655-656.

Phillipson, J.D. & Wright, C.W. 1991a. Antiprotozoal agents from plant sources. *Planta Medica* 57 (suppl.): 53-59.

Phillipson, J.D. & Wright, C.W. 1991b. Can ethnopharmacology contribute to the development of antimalarial agents? *Journal of Ethnopharmacology* 32: 155-165.

Phillipson, J.D., O'Neill, M.J., Wright, C.W., Bray, D.H. & Warhurst, D.C. 1987. Plants as sources of antimalarial and amoebicidal compounds. In: Leeuwenberg, A.J.M. (compilers). *Medicinal and Poisonous Plants of the Tropics*. Wageningen, Netherlands; Centre for Agricultural Publishing and Documentation. pp.70-79.

Spencer, C.F., Koniuszy, F.R. Rogers, E.F. Jr, Shavel, J., Easton, N.R., Kaczka, E.A. Jr, Kuehl, F.A., Phillips, R.F., Walti, A., Folkers, K., Malanga, C. & Seeler, A.O. 1947. Survey of plants for antimalarial activity. *Lloydia* 10: 145-174.

Bulgarian model for regulating the trade in plant material for medicinal and other purposes

D. Lange & M. Mladenova
Dr. Dagmar Lange, Jahnstr. 16, 71642 Ludwigsburg, Germany
Magdalena Mladenova, Bulgaria Agribusiness Centre, 3-A, 165 Street, Complex Izgreva, 1797 Sofia, Bulgaria

Introduction

The global importance of plants as a source of botanicals is enormous, a trade amounting to more than 300 thousand tonnes, and valued at more than US$ 800 million annually in 1995 and 1996 (Lange & Schippmann, 1997). Plants are the basis of a wide variety of goods ranging from food, phytopharmaceuticals, herbal remedies, perfumes, cosmetics, colouring agents, detergents, liqueurs, varnishes, fireworks, to detergents. The plant species dealt with in this paper are used in all the aforementioned categories, with the exception of food. Since, the term medicinal plant does not include all these different uses, the term botanical drug species is used by preference in this paper.

South-eastern and Eastern European countries are a rich source for botanical drug species within Europe. In a preliminary study by one of the authors (Lange,1996a), it was shown that these countries exported a total of about 11,000 tonnes annually to Germany during the period from 1991 to 1994 . This represented 30% of the average annual import to Germany, and 75% of all botanical drugs imported from the European countries. Within Eastern and South-eastern European countries, Bulgaria is the leading source country for Germany for botanical drugs, followed by Poland, Hungary, and Albania (Lange, 1996a). With regard to the global trade in botanical drugs, Bulgaria is eighth in the list of the leading countries of export, following after China, India, Germany, Singapore, Egypt, Chile, and the USA (Table 1). Thus trade in botanical drugs involving Bulgaria was the subject of an investigation conducted on behalf of the Federal Agency for Nature Conservation in Bonn and carried out in cooperation with the two authors.

Trade Structure in Bulgaria

Prior to the collapse of communism, botanical drugs were traded almost exclusively in Bulgaria by two state-controlled united cooperative enterprises. These were Bilkocoop and Bulgarcoop, which exported through their own foreign trade bureaus. During the last few years, the structure of trade has changed considerably. While the Bulgarian state has lost its monopoly, the two cooperative enterprises continue to operate and still remain the market leader. At the end of 1996, Bilkocoop became a part of Bulgarcoop. In addition, 50-60 smaller, private, mostly family-owned companies have become involved in the collecting, purchasing and export of botanical drugs.

Bilkocoop is also involved in the production of herbal and medicinal teas, at a volume of around 130 million tea-bags in 1995 mainly for the Bulgarian market. This company is also producing herbal bath additives, as well as different kinds of merchandise for the food industry, and supplies for pharmaceutical companies and pharmacies. Bilkocoop purchases the botanical drugs through other cooperatives distributed throughout the country, helps in cultivation of the plants, provides seeds and planting material, and guarantees to buy the agreed harvest.

Table 1: The 12 world leading countries of export of commodity group 1211. The countries are listed according to average export volumes corresponding to the years 1992-1995.

Country of export	Volume [tonnes]	Value lUSD 1,000]
China	121,900	264,500
India	32,600	45,950
Germany	14,400	68,500
Singapore	13,200	54,000
Egypt	11,250	12,350
Chile	11,200	23,500
USA	10,150	35,700
Bulgaria	7,800	11,000
Morocco	6,850	12,850
Mexico	6,300	9,300
Pakistan	4,800	3,300
France	4,700	26,300

Sources: (i) UNCTAD COMTRADE database, International Trade Centre, Geneva, Switzerland; ii) Foreign Trade Statistics of Bulgaria 1988-1996, National Statistic Institute, Sofia, Bulgaria (MLADENOVA, 1996).

The new private companies purchase a limited range of botanical drugs, mostly for export. Wild botanical drugs are collected by many people, mainly living in villages, who have a traditional knowledge of them. For many of the retired people in the country, collecting is a source of additional income, generally done sporadically and not according to a prior agreement. Because there is strong competition between the private companies and the cooperative enterprises a Private Herb Exchange has been established with similar tasks to those of Bilkocoop. It is also organising courses for the collectors.

Botanical drugs are sold mainly to larger wholesale drug traders abroad, sometimes backed by drug acencies, whereas direct sales from exporters to retail traders are an exception.

Volumes and Values

Every year more than 10,000 tonnes (estimated at 13,000-14,000 tonnes in 1995 and 1996) of botanical drugs are collected, purchased and processed in Bulgaria (Mladenova, 1996). Around 60-70% of the material is exported, while the other 30-40% remain in the country for the production of phytopharmaceuticals, herbal teas and spices.

From 1987 to 1995, the export of botanical drugs amounted to an average of 6,600 tonnes annually (Table 2). The annual export fluctuates considerably in this period:

between 1987 and 1989 it was around 5,000 tonnes, dropping to about 3,300 tonnes in 1990, probably because of the political changes in that time. In 1991 a sharp increase to more than 10,000 tonnes can be observed, however according to Mladenova (pers. comm.) it is likely, that this high volume is not correct. This is also indicated by the very high difference between the Bulgarian and the German Foreign Trade Statistics in 1991, amounting to 4,900 tonnes, which is much higher than in the following years (see below). Reasons can be again the changes in politics, and the change-over to the Harmonized System (HS, see below) in 1992. In 1993 5,100 tonnes have been exported. From 1994 onwards the export increased by far until 10,600 tonnes in 1995.

Germany is by far the most important purchaser for botanical drugs from Bulgaria. According to Bulgarian Foreign Trade Statistics, Germany imported on average more than 4,500 tonnes annually from 1987 to 1995 (table 2), that is on average 67% of the total Bulgarian export, with a distinct peak in 1991, when the import exceeded 8,500 tonnes. The German Foreign Trade Statistics reveals much lower import volumes from Bulgaria into Germany in the period 1991-1995 (Lange, 1996b), which are about 3,600 tonnes in 1991 (difference: 4,900 tonnes), 3,500 tonnes in 1992 (difference: 850 tonnes), 2,600 tonnes in 1993 (difference: 550 tonnes), 4,900 tonnes in 1994 (difference: 1,200 tonnes), and 6,472 tonnes in 1995 (difference: 500 tonnes).

In the list of the most important trading partners with Bulgaria in botanical drugs, Germany is followed by France, Spain, and Italy with imports of only 350-400 tonnes on average: that is less than 1/10th of Germany's imports. The only extra-European country with a noteworthy import of Bulgarian botanical drugs is the USA, which imports around 200 tonnes on average per annuum.

Little information is available on the export volumes of individual botanical drugs. The exports of botanical drugs are summarized mainly in one tariff code. From 1992 onwards, this has been Commodity Code No. 1211.90.00[1] , equivalent to the Harmonized System (HS), commonly accepted between GATT (General Agreement on Tariffs and Trade) members, which Bulgaria entered in 1996. As Bulgaria revealed individual trade figures for selected drugs until 1991, these are available for rose hips, linden flowers and leaves, peppermint, and chamomile (Mladenova, 1996). A further source for individual export volumes is the German Foreign Trade Statistics. Thus, in the German Utilisation Tariff some botanical drugs of high commercial value have been monitored separately since 1993 under the heading 1211.90. These include pyrethrum, mint, linden flowers and leaves, verbena, wild marjoram, and sage (Lange, 1996a). Wild thyme or serpolet, obtained from *Thymus serpyllum* s.l. is also monitored separately under the heading of spices (commodity group 0910.40.11). Additional information could be collected on the import/export of botanical drugs through a survey of traders.

According to the above sources, the most commonly exported commodity is mint, obtainted from peppermint *Mentha x piperita*, with the export to Germany increasing from 840 tonnes in 1993 to 2,350 tonnes in 1995. Other important products are linden flowers

---

"Plants and parts of plants (including seeds and fruits), of a kind used primarily in perfumery, in pharmacy or for insecticidal, fungicidal or similar purposes, fresh or dried, whether or not cut, crushed or powdered". An excerpt from the Harmonized Commodity Description and Coding System (HS) regarding commodity group 1211 is published in Lange & Schippmann (1997).

and leaves, obtained from small-leaved lime *Tilia cordata*, large-leaved lime *T. platyphyllos*, and silver lime *T. argentea* to be exported to Germany on an annual average of 280 tonnes since 1993, rose hips, collected from dog-rose *Rosa canina*, which have been exported from Bulgaria between 1987 and 1991 on an average of about 220 tonnes annually (Mladenova, 1996). Wild thyme or serpolet is exported from Bulgaria to Germany on average 18 tonnes annually from 1992-1995. Other botanical drugs exported in noteworthy volumes annually, but without exact trade figures, are common nettle (*Urtica dioica*), common balm (*Melissa officinalis*), valerian (*Valeriana officinalis*), lavender-blossom (*Lavandula angustifolia subsp. angustifolia*), St. John's Wort (*Hypericum perforatum*), savory (*Satureja hortensis*), chamomile (*Matricaria recutita*), black elder-blossom (*Sambucus nigra*), yarrow (*Achillea millefolium*), betony (*Stachys officinalis*), common dandelion (*Taraxacum offininalis*), and the fruits of hawthorn (*Crataegus spp.*), bilberry (*Vaccinium myrtillus*), common juniper (*Juniperus communis*), horse-chestnut (*Aesculus hippocastanum*), and dwarf elder (*Sambucus ebulus*).

The value of the exported botanical drugs amounted to USD 9.4 million in 1992, and increased from USD 7 million in 1993 to USD 15.4 million in 1995. This correspondend to an average export price of USD 1.40 per kilogram.

Compared to exports, the imported volume of botanical drugs into Bulgaria is very low. From 1992-1995 Bulgaria imported on average 400 tonnes annually. Altogether, imports came from 13 different countries during this period. However, in 1992 (520 tonnes) and 1993 (300 tonnes) these came mainly from Turkey, and in 1994 (240 tonnes) and 1995 (350 tonnes) from Macedonia. The value of the imported merchandise fluctuates between USD 0,7 and 1 million.

There is no information available on the individual botanical drugs that are imported. But according to Mladenova (1996), in the last 2-3 years rose hips have been imported, mainly from Russia, Albania, and Macedonia. These imports have been destined mainly for re-exports. In addition, some botanical drugs, which are not native to or cultivated in Bulgaria, or are not available in sufficient quantities are imported. These include the flower calyces of red sorrel, for example, which are a component of herbal teas, and the herb of periwinkle (*Catharanthus roseus*) produced in phytopharmaceuticals. Other botanical drugs, such as the bark of alder buckthorn (*Frangula alnus*) and the leaves of bearberry (*Arctostaphylos uva-ursi*) have been imported for the Bulgarian market, since the collection of and trade in these have been subject to restrictions. This is also true for the flowers of sandy immortelles (*Helichrysum arenarium*).

Botanical Drug Supply

Botanical drug species are one of the natural resources of Bulgaria (Hardalova, 1997), and collecting them has a long tradition. Around 750 plant species, that is 21% of the 3,567 vascular plants of Bulgaria, are used in folk medicine, in the food and pharmaceutical industry, and for export. Of these 200 to 300 species are the most commonly used (Hardalova, 1997). More than two thirds are known to be exported to Germany (Lange, 1996b). Most of the species are collected in the wild, and an estimated 20-25% are produced from cultivation (Hardalova, 1997). Important cultivated plant species are peppermint (*Mentha x piperita*), rose hips (*Rosa canina*), valerian (*Valeriana officinalis*), chamomile *(Matricaria recutita)*, marsh-mallow *(Althaea officinalis)*, and milk thistle *(Silybum marianum)*.

Table 2: Exports volumes from Bulgaria for commodity group 1211. The countries are listed according to average export volumes corresponding to the years 1987-1995, arranged according to average volume.

Country of export	1987	1988	1989	1990	1991	1992	1993	1994	1995
Germany	3,185	3,949	2,569	2,233	8,586	4,334	3,134	6,135	6,975
Spain	235	206	958	299	147	440	317	493	472
France	321	416	830	382	307	301	357	271	364
Italy	317	223	154	189	219	423	425	754	620
USA	161	181	122	59	129	163	271	304	532
Switzerland	140	84	32	44	138	220	248	229	271
Austria	67	116	179	126	111	229	91	145	69
Greece	10	20	10	-	91	52	30	284	399
Sweden	190	133	190	20	276	36	-	-	-
Poland	-	-	-	-	-	4	10	209	483
Hungary	-	-	-	-	-	-	47	50	209
Netherlands	88	37	-	-	7	6	38	27	52
Belgium	-	87	-	-	-	43	21	44	-
Turkey	-	-	-	-	-	53	19	10	35
Argentina	-	-	-	-	-	45	48	-	-
Macedonia	-	-	-	-	-	-	36	24	-
Ireland	-	-	-	-	-	-	20	-	43
Czech Republic	-	-	-	-	27	15	4	-	-
England	-	-	-	-	-	-	-	31	11
Finland	-	-	-	-	-	-	-	30	12
Yugoslavia	-	-	38	-	-	2	-	-	-
Croatia	-	-	-	-	-	-	-	-	20
Russia	-	-	-	-	-	-	-	-	19
Jordan	-	-	-	-	-	-	-	-	15
Romania	-	-	-	-	-	-	-	-	5
Georgia	-	-	-	-	-	-	-	-	5
Slovenia	-	-	-						2
Total	4,710	5,454	5,110	3,358	10,042	6,440	5,139	9,052	10,601

Volumes are given in tonnes.

Source: Foreign Trade Statistics of Bulgaria 1988-1996, National Statistic Institute, Sofia, Bulgaria (MLADENOVA, 1996).

As a result of the high percentage of wild-collected plant material that is used and the huge volumes collected every year, there is a high risk of damaging, or even destroying the natural resources of Bulgaria's botanical drug species. According to Hardalova (1997) 20% of wild botanical drug species are weeds or occur in rural habitats, and are not threatened by collection. However, for the remaining species a permanent means of control, or even restictive measures, are necessary.

Legislation

The trade in, to and from Bulgaria in botanical drugs is governed by legislation at national and international levels. Those species protected internationally are covered in the Convention on International Trade with Endangered Species of Wild Flora and Fauna (CITES). Those protected nationally are listed (i) in the Bulgarian Ordinance on the Conservation of Species, and/or (ii) are subject to legal restrictions and ordinances concerning control of utilization and trade of the botanical drug species. In addition, botanical drug species can be protected through habitat protection.

While no species used as a source for a botanical drug is listed in CITES Appendix I, eight species are listed in CITES Appendix II: snowdrop (*Galanthus nivalis*), pyramidal orchid (*Anacamptis pyramidalis*), butterfly orchid (*Orchis papilionacea*), globose orchid (*O. globosa*), military orchid (*O. militaris*), Provence orchid (*O. provincialis*), *Cyclamen coum*, and ivy-leaved sowbread (*C. hederifolium*).

The Bulgarian Species Conservation Legislation came into force on 21.7.1989 (Ordinance No. 718, dated 20.6.1989). This ordinance updated the first list of protected plant species published in 1961, and covers 330 plant species. Criteria for inclusion in this listing are varied, including over-exploitation, limited natural distribution, habitat destruction and difficulties with dissemination (Hardalova, 1997). For all the 330 plant species, cutting, collecting, picking, uprooting, trading, exporting them, either as fresh or as dried material is stricty forbidden. Additionally, it is prohibited to harvest their seeds, bulbs, or other reproductive organs. Amongst the 330 plant species, thirty-seven species are used for medicinal or related purposes. Examples for protected species with a narrow distribution in Bulgaria are: Round-leaved sundew (*Drosera rotundifolia*), liquorice (*Glycyrrhiza glabra*), Rhapontic rhubarb (*Rheum rhaponticum*), common rue (*Ruta graveolens*), sideritis (mountain tea) (*Sideritis scardica*), and yew (*Taxus baccata*). A species which is protected because of over-exploitation is yellow gentian (*Gentiana lutea*), for example, and species who are are affected by habitat destruction are sweet-flag (*Acorus calamus*), bogbean (*Menyanthes trifoliata*), and different Orchis-species (Hardalova, 1997).

According to Hardalova (1997) a total of 820 ha of conservation sites exist in Bulgaria for the protection of botanical drug species around 50 protected areas. They have been established to protect the habitat of summer snowflake (*Leucojum aestivum*), peony (*Paeonia peregrina*), liquorice (*Glycyrrhiza glabra*), snowdrop (*Galanthus nivalis*), elecampane (*Inula helenium*), and cowslip (*Primula veris*), inter alia. The collection of these species is forbidden. In addition to this in-situ conservation, about 150 botanical drug species are preserved in collections of living plants and seeds of the Academy of Sciences.

Trade in botanical drugs in Bulgaria is subject to different laws and regulations established in 1991 under the Law for the Protection of the Environment (Mladenova, 1996). In addition to taxes and duties, import/export turnover taxes, excise taxes, any customs duties, possible countervailing duties, regulations concerning required documents for imports/exports, or registration and transaction charges, there are some interesting legal requirements, which are described below:

(A) Where botanical drug species occur in the forests, they come under the jurisdiction of the Forestry Committee, and their use is subject to forestry laws, which the Forestry Administration is responsible for applying (Hardalova, 1997). In the forests, wild-collecting is seen as a business and thus fees have to be paid for using the so-called forestry by-products. The rates are species-specific and are paid in leva per kilogram (Decree No. 202 dated 26.9.1994, published in Official Gazette No. 82, 1994), but charges will only apply when forestry resources are exploited commercially. For example, the charge for 1 kg of the roots of cowslip *(Primula veris)* is 4 leva, and for leaves of ribwort plantain (*Plantago lanceolata*) 2.50 leva must be paid. For further examples see table 3.

Table 3: Examples for botanical drugs collected in the forests in Bulgaria and the charges to be paid for their commercial use. - Source: MLADENOVA (1996).

Common name	Scientific name	Plant part used	Charge [leva/kg]
Hazel	*Coryllus avellana*	bark	3,00
Hazel	*Coryllus avellana*	leaves	1,50
Bilberry	*Vaccinium myrtillus*	leaves	2,50
Bilberry	*Vaccinium myrtillus*	fruits	6,00
Wild strawberry	*Fragaria vesca*	leaves	2,50
Wild thyme, serpolet	*Thymus serpyllum*	herb	1,50
St. John's Wort	*Hypericum perforatum*	herb	1,50
Hawthorn	*Cratuegus monogyna*	fruits	3,00
Black elder	*Sambucus nigra*	flowers	1,50
Orange mullein	*Verbascum phlomoides*	leaves	1,50
Cowslip	*Primula veris*	flowers	2,00
Cowslip	*Primula veris*	roots	4,00
Dog-rose	*Rosa canina*	fruits	3,00
Large-leaved lime	*Tilia platyphyllos*	flowers	2,00
Mistletoe	*Viscum album*	leaves	1,50
Ribwort plantain	*Plantago lanceolata*	leaves	2,50
Common dandelion	*Taraxacum officinalis*	herb	1,50
Common dandelion	*Taraxacam officinalis*	roots	4,00

Explanation: Herb, i.e. the aerial part of the plant. - 1 DM = 1,000 leva (1.7.1997), 1USD = 1,800 lava.

(B) Several fees are collected by the Ministry of Environment for the National Fund for Protection of the Environment. Those are related to the granting of import/export certificates (lastest Decree No. 132 dated 31.3.1997, published in Official Gazette No. 28, 3.3.1997). Because of the high rate of inflation, the system of setting charges changed in 1997 from a fixed amount (for 1996) to fees determined as percentage of the minimal monthly wage in Bulgaria (April 1997: 29,920 leva, May 1997: 41,290 leva). The following are charges for the export of each wild-collected species: (i) to export a plant species not covered by any regulations 5% (1996: 50 levas), for those which are subject to species conservation regulations 10% (1996: 200 levas); (ii) the rate for the export of a wild plant species that has been cultivated is 2%; (iii) the fee for operating a purchasing centre for botanical drug species, inter alia, amounts to 30% (1996: 500 leva); (iv) to export a Bulgarian species included in CITES, the charge is 45% (1996: 1,000 levas), and to export, import or re-export a foreign species included in CITES the charge is 75% (1996: 1,500 levas); (v) For the allocation of quotas for using threatened biological resources 10% (1996: 200 levas) for each species is charged (see paragraph C).

(C) Since 1991, wild-harvesting of, and trade in, threatened botanical drug species are subject to restrictions and prohibitions, issued by the Ministry of the Environment. Several ordinances regulate the gathering, trade and export of selected wild botanical drug species, with the aim of protecting them and their natural habitats, to re-establish wild populations, and to encourage cultivation of some species (Ordinance No. RD-48, dated 15.2.1995, published in Official Gazette No. 21, 28.2.1995, added by Ordinance No. RD-50, dated 17.2.1995, published in Official Gazette No. 22, 7.3.1995, revised with Ordinance No. RD-76, dated 28.2.1996, published in Continent, dated 8.3.1996, and Ordinance No. RD-97, dated 28.3.1997). These ordinances establish restrictions and prohibitions on collecting, trading and exporting botanical drug species:

(i) At least 14 plant species are totally prohibited from being collected from the wild, traded and processed for commercial purposes (table 4). Thus, the species, marsh-mallow (*Althaea officinalis)*, madder (*Rubia tinctorium)*, valerian (*Valeriana officinalis)*, inter alia, must be cultivated for commercial use.

(ii) The collecting of 23 other plant species from the wild, their processing, and trade are subject to restrictions. A quota-system was established for these species. The volumes of each species (according to plant parts used) which can be collected from their natural habitats in the different Bulgarian districts, and which are allowed to be exported have been published in the Official Gazette every spring since 1992, drawn up by specialists of the Ministry of Environment, and the Institute of Botany. The list of plant species affected by this order has been modified slightly, but the volumes which are allowed to be gathered vary considerably from year to year according to the species and the region. Table 4 lists the species concerned, table 5 shows examples for quotas for botanical drugs allowed to be collected by region in 1997.

(iii) The export of six additional botanical drugs collected from the wild is strictly prohibited. These include the herb (aerial parts) of summer snowflake (*Leucojum aestivum)*, the bark of alder buckthorn (*Frangula alnus)*, and the roots of cowslip (*Primula veris*)(table 4).

The following is an illustration of the quota-system:

- In 1995, and 1996, quotas for 18 botanical drugs obtained from 15 of the 23 plant species mentioned in table 4, column 2, have been set up, whereas in 1997, quotas for 19 botanical drugs obtained from 15 plant species have been published. Collecting of the remaining botanical drugs, viz. plant species from the wild, as well as trading or processing them for commercial purposes has been prohibited.

Example 1: In 1995 and 1996 it was totally prohibited to collect the roots of deadly nightshade *(Atropa bella-donna)* from the wild, however 2,550 kg are allowed in 1997 (table 5).

Example 2: The herb of asarabacca *(Asarum europaeum)* was not permitted to be obtained from the wild in 1995, but in 1996 (500 kg) and 1997 (50 kg, see table 5).

- This ordinance includes an annual periodic ban on the exploitation of regional populations. It was forbidden to collect any wild plant species involved in the districts Pazardgik, Silistra, and Smolian in 1995, the districts Dobrich, Kardjali, and Jambol in 1996, and the districts Lovech, and again Dobrich, Kardjali, Silistra, and Smolian in 1997.
- From year to year the total and the regional quotas for each species have changed.

Example 1: In 1996 and 1997 collection of 500 kg Herba Adonidis (aerial part of yellow pheasant's eye *Adonis vernalis*) in Razgrad district was allowed (table 5), where it was forbidden in 1995.

Example 2: Wild-collecting of a total of 3,700 kg of Folia Belladonnae, obtained from the leaves of deadly nightshade *(Atropa bella-donna)*, was allowed in 1995, and the whole volume was allowed to be exported, whereas in 1996 and 1997 6,050 kg respectively 4,320 kg were allowed to be wild-harvested. Only half of the volume, however, was destined for export (table 5).

Example 3: In 1995 it was forbidden to collect the leaves of bearberry *(Arctostaphylos uva-ursi)* from natural habitats. In 1996 it was allowed to collect 800 kg in Pazardgik district only, and in 1997 the quota is 2,500 kg shared to Blagoevgrad district 1,000 kg, and to Pazardjk 1,500 kg.

Example 4: In 1995 the quota for the flowers of cowslip (*Primula veris*) was 6,300 kg. In 1996 it increased up to 12,000 kg, and dropped in 1997 to 8,670 kg (table 5).

The Ministry of Environment, the Forestry Committee, and the local Authorities are responsible for administering the control. The quota-system described is based on scientific research done by specialists of the Ministry of Environment in cooperation with the Institute of Botany of the Bulgarian Academy of Science, and the National Centre of Phytotherapy and Popular Medicine. Regional Environmental Inspectorates approved by regional Forestry Administrations are responsible for allocation of the quantities of the wild-harvested botanical drugs in each country. Purchaser of these plants must make their applications by the end of the previous year. The botanical drugs affected by these ordinances must to be accompanied by documents of origin up to the end user. Those obtained from cultivation, are not subject to prohibitions and restrictions. However, this must be substantiated by documents from the Municpality, State Forestries, and regional Environmental Inspectorates.

For controlling the legal requirements of the ordinances mentioned, the purchasers of the botanical drugs involved are obliged (i) to register with the regional Environmental Inspectorates, (ii) to ensure complete access to the controlling authorities, and (iii) to keep the necessary documentation for all transactions concerning these botanical drugs.

Table 4: Botanical drug species affected by the prohibitions and restrictions on collecting, trading and exporting.

Total prohibition of collecting, trade, and processing from the wild, for commercial purposes	Restrictions on collecting, trade, and processing from the wild, for commercial purposes (quota system)	Prohibition of export
Flowering plants		
Althaea officinalis	*Adonis vernalis*	*Atropa bella-donna* (roots)
Artemisia santonicam	*Alchemilla vulgaris s.*1.	*Berberis vulgaris* (bark)
Cnicus benedictus	*Allium ursinum*	*Leucojum arstivum* (herb)
Convallaria majalis	*Angelica pancicii1*	*Paeonia peregrina* (tuber)
Glaucium flavum	*Arctostaphylos uva-ursi*	*Primula veris* (roots)
Helichrysum arenariarn	*Artemisia alba*	*Frangula alaus* (bark)
Inula helenium	*Asarum europaeum*	*Stachys officinalis* (roots)
Orchis spp.	*Atropa bella-donna*	
Origanum vulgare subsp. *hirtum*2	*Berberis vulgaris*	
Rubia tinctorium	*Carlina acanthifolia*	
*Salvia tomentosa*3	*Gallum odoratum*	
Valeriana officinalis	*Hyssopus officinalis*	
	Leucojum aestivum	
	Paeonia peregrina	
	Primula veris	
	Frangula alaus	
	Ruscus aculentus	
	Sedum acre	
	Stachys officinalis	
	Vinca minor	
Conifers		
-	*Juniperus oxycedrus*	
Ferns		
Aspleniarn trichomanes		
Asplenium scolopendrium		
Lichens		
-	*Cetraria islandica*	
Algae		
-	*Cystoseira barbata*	

The nomenclature of the vascular plants is according to Flora Europaea (Tutin, T.G. & al., 1968-1993).
1 =A. *sylvestris;* 2 = *o heracleoticum;* 3 =S. *officinalis;*

Source: Ordinance No. RD-48 of 1995, Ordinance No. RD-50 of 1995, Ordinance No. RD-76 of 1996, and Ordinance No. RD-97 of 1997.

When comparing the quota-tables of 1995-1997, it could be stated that the overall volume of botanical drugs, affected by the ordinances mentioned, fluctuates only between 73.5 tonnes in 1995, 77 tonnes in 1996, and around 62.4 tonnes in 1997. However the share of the botanical drugs directed to the internal Bulgarian market only, increased from 5% in 1995 to 28% in 1997.

Table 5: Examples for quotas for botanical drugs allowed to be collected by region in 1997. - Source: Ordinance No. RD-97, dated 28.3.1997.

District	*Asarum europaeum*	*Primula veris*		*Atropa bella-donna*		*Arctostaphylos uva-ursi*	*Adonis vernalis*
Part of plant used	herb	flowers	roots	leaves	roots	leaves	herb
Blagoevgrad	-	800	15	300	-	1,000	-
Varna	-	-	-	-	-	-	700
V. Tirnova	-	500	-	300	-	-	50
Vidin	-	-	-	700	--	-	-
Vratza	-	800	-	200	-	-	-
Gabrovo	50	500	100	500	50	-	50
Kustendil	-	400	-	-	-	-	-
Montana	-	700	-	500	-	-	100
Pazardjik	-	-	-	-	1,000	1.500	-
Pernik	-	500	-	-	-	-	600
Pleven	-	300	-	300	-	-	-
Plovdiv	-	-	-	-	-	-	-
Razgrad	-	500	-	-	-	-	500
Ruse	-	500	-	-	-	-	200
Sliven	-	800	200	500	-	-	-
Sofia	-	20	-	20	-	-	-
St. Zagora	-	800	200	1,000	1,500	-	-
Targoviste	-	250	-	-	-	-	500
Schumen	-	800	-	-	-	-	500
Jambol	-	500	200	-	-	-	-
Total [kg]	50	8,670	715	4,320	2,550	2,500	3,200
Internal market only [kg]	50	1,000	715	2.000	2,550	2,500	500

Conclusion

Demand for certain botanical drugs is expected to increase (Mladenova, 1996). This is not only true for cultivated species, like peppermint (*Mentha x piperita*), common balm (*Melissa officinalis*), or chamomile (*Matricaria recutita*), but also for some wild species used as raw material for herbal and medicinal teas, as well as for the production in Bulgaria of phytopharmaceuticals and of cosmetics, such as creams and shampoos.

The laws and regulations concerning wild-collection of some of the highly-sought-after botanical drug species, will enforce an increase in their cultivation. Further, according to Mladenova (1996), the share of the cultivated plant material to be exported will increase in the future.

The Bulgarian model for controlling and protecting botanical drug species includes not only species and habitat conservation measurements, but also legislation on the collection and trade of some selected species. In this respect, it is unique. However legislation and regulation alone are insufficient to achieve the sustainable use of the species concerned. Additional administrative, technological and educational measures to the purchasers, growers or collectors will need to be established (Hardalova , 1997). An unintended, however, negative consequence of the legislation concerning control of utilization and trade of the botanical drug species could be that botanical drug traders and producers of herbal teas, phytopharmaceuticals or cosmetics will get around Bulgaria's law by purchasing raw materials abroad. As stated above, this has been observed for some species during recent years. As a result, these species could become scarce in other countries. Consequently, it will be necessary to ensure that imports of those particular botanical drugs are also subject to control, or even to restrictions, in cooperation with the source countries. Thus, there is a need to develop guidelines for the sustainable exploitation of wild plant resources, including requirements for the qualifications of those involved in the trade.

Further scientific research is warranted on cultivation, development of population status due to habitat change and exploitation, type of harvesting, and the demands of the plant species in the market. All of these measures should be taken into account with regard to the expected increased demand for botanical drug species within the coming years.

Acknowledgements

Both authors would like to express their gratitude to staff members of the Scientific Authorities of CITES, Bonn, namely Natalie Hofbauer, Uwe Schippmann and Hajo Schmitz-Kretschmer, and of the Agribusiness Centre of the Institute of Trade, especially to Milena Nalbantova doing the translation from Bulgarian to English, and Desisslava Georgieva for the data processing. Also, we would like to thank Rayna Hardalova from the Ministry of Environment who supported the project with her knowledge and provided the official documents.

References

Hardalova, R. (1997): The use of medicinal plants in Bulgaria and their protection. - Proceedings of Planta Europa, 2-8 September 1995, Hyères, France 184-187.

Lange, D. (1996a): Untersuchungen zum Heilpflanzenhandel in Deutschland. Ein Beitrag zum internationalen Artenschutz. - 130 pp.; Bundesamt fur Naturschutz, Bonn.

Lange, D. (1996b): Der Handel mit drogenliefernden Pflanzenarten zwischen Deutschland und Bulgarien. - In: D. Lange, Analyse der Gefährdung von Heilpflanzen durch den internationalen Handel: 50-110. - unpublished report for the Federal Agency for Nature Conservation in Bonn, Germany, 1996.

Lange, D. & Schippmann, U. (1997). Trade Survey of Medicinal Plants in Germany A Contribution to International Plant Species Conservation. Bonn-Bad Godesberg (Bundesamt für Naturschutz) 128pp. Annexes (pp.I-XVI).

Mladenova, M. (1996): The trade in medicinal plants between Germany and Bulgaria. - Bulgarian Agri-business Centre; Sofia (unpublished report).

Phytomedicinal forest harvest in the United States

James A. Duke
Botanical Consultant, Herbal Vineyard, Inc
8210 Murphy Rd; Fulton MD 20759; USA
Fax: ++ 1 301 498 5738 Email: jimduke@cpcug.org

Abstract*

The Appalachian deciduous forests have been and continue to be a major source of some minor and major phytomedicinals in the southeastern United States. Fortunately, many important medicinal species are rather weedy and not at all endangered. Indeed massive biological control programs have contained e.g. *Hypericum perforatum* in the western US. Some American species may have been diminished by medicinal plant collecting, e.g. species in the genera *Aristolochia, Cypripedium, Echinacea, Hydrastis, Panax* and the like, and several species from the Orchidaceae family. Uses and abundance of some of the native US forest medicinal plant species and weedy invaders are discussed. As with legitimate medicines, herbal medicines are sometimes overplayed (Herbal hype) or intentionally misrepresented (Herbal hoax), with serious implications on their resource availability. Many of the phytomedicinal compounds are widely distributed, either taxonomically or geographically. Biologically active alkaloid's, like: berberine, sanguinarine, arbutin and pulegone are widely occurring in the plant kingdom. Substitution or even competition among some medicinal plants from different parts of the world might have serious impacts on the present and future resource status of these species as is demonstrated for the case of Chinese-, American-, and Siberian ginseng.

Introduction: resource availability

Fortunately, many important medicinal species are rather weedy and not at all endangered. Indeed massive biological control programs have targeted and, to a degree, reduced infestations of *Hypericum perforatum*, under the name "klamath weed", in the western US. In 1997, under the name "Saint John's-wort", this species became the top selling herbal medicine for its antidepressant activity. Several species of *Hypericum* contain the antiretroviral compound hypericin. Pokeweed, *Phytolacca americana*, is the only source of the antiviral Pokeweed Antiviral Mitogen, which can be delivered to target sites on monoclonal antibodies. For its new Designer Food cancer-preventive program, the late Herb Pierson was looking at a pair of weeds, the garlic-mustard *(Alliaria petiolata* [M. Bieb.] Cavara & Grande), which may combine the activities and phytochemicals of the garlic and mustard families, e.g., respectively allincin and sulforaphane, and the burdock *(Arctium spp.),* an ingredient in two noteworthy "anticancer formulae", the Hoxsey

* This chapter is based on an earlier and unpublished draft by Dr. J. Duke, which has been made available in collaboration with Judi DuCellier, Andrea Ottesen, Peggy Duke, and Ed Claflin, of Rodale Press, who allowed to reuse some of the illustrations made by Peggy Duke from 'The Green Pharmacy" (Rodale Press, 1997).

Formula and the Essiac Formula. Burdock is well endowed with medicinal lignans that might help in Hodgkin's disease. All four of these weeds occur on my 6 acre farmette 20 miles southwest of Baltimore. The Designer Food Programme was also looking closely at licorice, *Glycyrrhiza glabra*, which is a serious weed, e.g. in Turkish wheat fields. Parallel biological activities will probably be demonstrated by America's *Glycyrrhiza lepidota*, not yet really a weed.

It is hard for me to call the mayapple *(Podophyllum peltatum)* a weed, but it is certainly a common woodland "wild flower". Podophyllotoxin was one "Drug of Choice" for brain tumors and Hodgkin's disease. Recently we have witnessed the advent of the semisynthetic etoposide (a modification of the molecule of podophyllotoxin). In 1984 and 1986 it was approved for cancer of the testicles and small cell lung cancer, respectively. Long before we knew about etoposide and/or vepeside, there was an American market for one hundred tons of mayapple rhizome, mostly for use as a cathartic. It was even a component of the famous Carter's Little Liver Pills. For years, the resin podophyllin from the rhizome was the drug of choice for venereal warts (condyloma acuminatum). Yet at a Symposium on Plant Life in South Asia, I heard Tony Nasir complain that *Podophyllum hexandxum* had all but been eliminated from Pakistan forests by an occidental drug company developing etoposide. Fortunately, it has been brought under cultivation in the hill country of Pakistan. Like our species, it is a bit recalcitrant from seed, but rhizome transplants are easy. If for some reason, Asian trade in *Podophyllum hexandrum* were discontinued, much greater collection pressure on our American species can be predicted. According to Principe (1989), etoposide already has annual sales of ca $15 million in the late 1980s but by now, sales are estimated to have topped $400 million a year. Thus economically, *Podophyllum* has challenged and exceeded the Madagascar periwinkle, *Catharanthus roseus*, the number 1 antileukemic plant. Products derived from the periwinkle had a wholesale value of $35 million in 1977 which Principe (1989) suggests would have translated to a retail value of $140 million.

The Appalachian deciduous forests have been and continues to be a major source of some minor and major phytomedicinals in the southeastern United States. Established adventives and Native American medicinal species still harvested today include: *Achillea millefolium* (yarrow), *Acorus calamus* (sweetflag), *Arctium* spp (burdock), *Asarum canadense* (wild ginger), *Dioscorea* spp. (wild yam), *Echinacea* spp. (coneflower), *Hamamelis virginiana* (witch hazel), *Hydrastis canadensis* (goldenseal), *Hypericum* spp. (St John's-wort), *Lobelia inflata* (Indian tobacco), *Lycopodium* spp. (club moss), *Oenothera biennis* (evening primrose), *Panax quinquefolius* (ginseng), *Passiflora incarnate* (passion fruit), *Phytolacca americana* (pokeweed), *Pinus strobus* (white pine), *Plantago major* (plantain), *Podophyllum peltatum* (mayapple), *Prunella vulgaris* (heal-all), *Prunus serotina* (black cherry), *Rumex crispus* (yellow dock), *Salix* spp. (willow), *Sanguinaria canadensis* (bloodroot), *Sassafras albidum* (sassafras), *Smilax* spp. (sarsaparilla), and *Veratrum viride* (hellebore).

Markets have existed for others now or in the past decade, e.g. species of *Adiantum, Agrimonia, Alnus, Aplectrum, Aralia, Arctostaphylos, Aristolochia, Apocynum, Artemisia, Berberis, Cassia, Caulophyllum, Chimaphila, Cimicifuga, Collinsonia, Cypripedium, Dryopteris, Equisetum, Euonymus, Eupatorium, Filipendula, Frangula, Gaultheria,*

Geranium, Glechoma, Hedeoma, Humulus, Hydrangea, Juglans, Juniperus, Lactuca, Medicago, Melilotus, Mentha, Mitchella, Myrica, Nepeta, Polygala, Polygonatum, Polygonum, Quercus, Rhus, Sambucus, Scutellaria, Senecio, Solidago, Spigelia, Stellaria, Tanacetum, Taraxacum, Tephrosia, Teucrium, Tipularia, Trifolium, Trilisa, Ulmus, Verbascum, Verbena, Veronicastrum and *Zanthoxylum*.

However, some American species may have been diminished by medicinal plant collecting, e.g. species in the *genera Aristolochia, Cypripedium, Echinacea, Hydrastis, Panax* and the like. *Sanguinaria* could be, unless the Food and Drug Administration lands on a toothpaste manufacturer, reportedly using sanguinarine in its antiplaque toothpaste. American medicinal usage may have contributed to the decimation of *Cephaelis* ("ipecac") in Latin America, *Rauvolfia serpentina* ("Indian snakeroot") in India, *Podophyllum hexandrum* (" Himalayan mayaple") in India and Pakistan, *Tabebuia* spp ("pau d'arco") and *Uncaria tomentosa* ("cat's claw") in South America. After a cancer scare re *Rauvolfia*, more than a decade ago, it looked as though there might be pressure on America's *Veratrum viride* as an alternative source of tranquilizers. (There are four *Veratrum's* proposed for listing as endangered of threatened, DOI, 1985). The crunch on *Veratrum* never came, as the cancer alarm re *Rauvolfia* was later rescinded. Alternative sources of reserpine exist in other species of Rauvolfia in Africa and Latin America. India has proposed CITES protection for both *Rauvolfia serpentine* and *Podophyllum hexandrum* (Marshall, 1989).

America's long courtship with sedatives and tranquilizers may have decimated ladyslipper populations here and there. Once known in Europe as American valerian, the ladyslipper has a long history as an antispasmodic, sedative and tranquilizer. The herb industry is attempting to help preserve ladyslippers. Many of the bigger dealers have publicly announced that they no longer deal in ladyslippers (McCaleb, 1990). North Carolina herbalists are attempting to propagate ladyslippers in tissue culture in hopes of mastering their cultivation, much as they have mastered ginseng cultivation.

Ladyslipper is not the only orchid endangered by medicinal collectors. One Baltimore herbalist told me he could get $18 for the paired tubers of *Aplectrum* or *Tipularia*. Like the middle eastern "salep", paired tubers of these species suggest the testicles and hence, following the "Doctrine of Signatures", they are promoted as "aphrodisiac". Indeed the family Orchidaceae may owe its name to the testicle-like tubers.

Availability of similar active plant components amoung different species

In a languishing unpublished draft I have, called "Gaia's Galenicals", I note that many of the phytomedicinal compounds, e.g. allicin, aloe-emodin, anabasine, arbutin, atropine, berberine, caffeine, capsaicin, chrysarobin, colchicine, dopa, emetine, ephedrine, eugenol, gossypol, harmaline, hypericin, lobeline, menthol, nicotine, podophyllotoxin, quercetin, quercitrin, quinine, reserpine, rutin, salicylic acid, sanguinarine, scopolamine, sitosterol, theophylline, trigonelline, xanthotoxin, and yohimbine, are widely distributed, either taxonomically or geographically. On the other hand, some of our abused phytomedicinals have a relatively narrow taxonomic base, cocaine limited to the genus *Erythroxylum*, codeine, morphine and thebaine limited largely to the genus *Papaver*, and THC

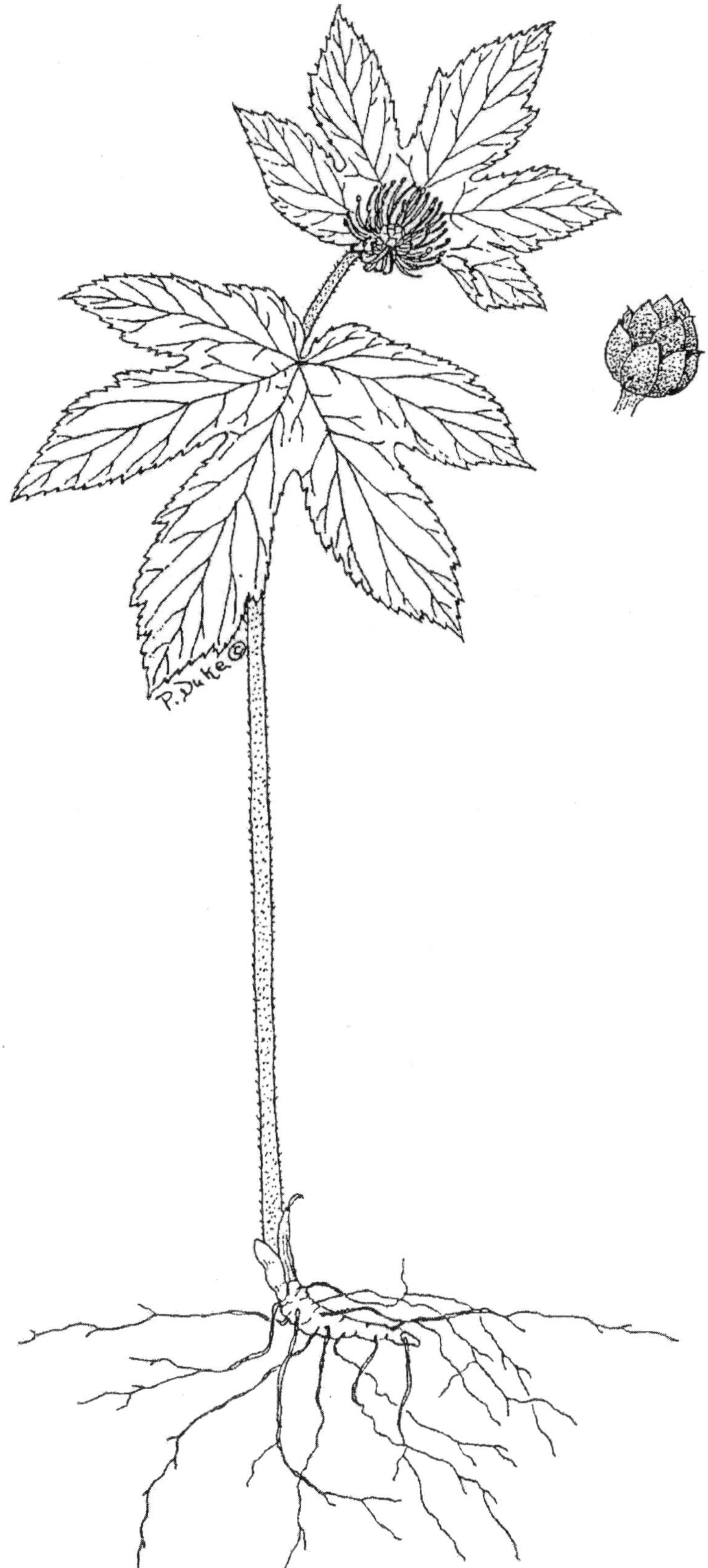

Figure 1: Goldenseal (*Hydrastis canadensis*)

(tetrahydrocannabinol) to *Cannabis*. It is a sad commentary that the US spends $150 billion on illicit drugs while the world spends $150 billion on legitimate prescription drugs.

The first major big-buck event that involved a forest medicinal was with the wild yam, *Dioscorea villosa*, well endowed with disogenin. Wisely, chemist Dr. Russell Marker, back in the forties, realized that all the major expensive hormones could be synthesized from the readily available starter material diosgenin. I have two sources of disogenin, the phytochemical to which the steroid and contraceptive industries owe their meteoric ascent in the 1940s and 1950s, *Dioscorea villosa* and *Smilax* spp., growing native in my east temperate forest area. In our folklore, there has evolved a belief that the wild yam is more useful for females, the sarsaparilla more useful for males. In Moerman's (1986) excellent and authoritative book, Medicinal Plants of Native America, only one use is cited for *Dioscorea villosa*, for the relief of pain during childbirth. The macho "Carrion Flower" is used for afterbirth, backache, body odor, boils, constipation, cramps, dysmenorrhea, gastrosis, hoarseness, nephrosis, pain, and pulmonosis. Not only do the yams contain sapogenins, they contain some 100-1,000 ppms sterols, mostly beta-sitosterol (Spiller, 1996). Sixty milligrams a day of sitosterol is reportedly efficacious in the old man's prostate ailment, benign prostatic hyperplasia or hypertrophy (BPH). The literature, erroneously, attributes progesterone (and more recently DHEA) to *Dioscorea* and testosterone to *Smilax*. In building my Father Natures Farmacy database (Duke, 1992a,b), I find no legitimate reports of those hormones in these plants. Plant extracts may have occasionally been spiked with many different hormones, and there is no doubt that many so-called wild yam creams are spiked with progesterone and some are spiked with DHEA. Over the years, the starter material of choice became soybean, as first the North American yam and then the Mexican yam priced themsevles out of business. Still today there is brisk trade in the forest species, *Dioscorea villosa*, for natural wild yam creams, being widely promoted for hormonal balancing problems. Soon, it may become as endangered here as the Asian *Dioscorea's*, overharvested, e.g., in India

Herbal hype and herbal hoax: the case of goldenseal, bloodroot, coneflower and pennyroyal

As with legitimate medicines, herbal medicines are sometimes overplayed (Herbal hype) or intentionally misrepresented (Herbal hoax). Like ginseng, goldenseal *(Hydrastis canadensis.)* has locally been over collected. Current pressures on goldenseal may partially result from an Herbal hoax, the widely spread untruth that goldenseal could help mask illicit drugs in urinalysis. More pressure may have been generated by testimonials of women who experienced remissions of uterine cancers while or after taking goldenseal. Granted, goldenseal does contain the biologically active alkaloid, berberine, which has several legitimate uses, and which has proven antitumor activity, in vitro at least. But berberine is widely occurring in the plant kingdom, including some much more common weeds, and some even rarer than the goldenseal. Berberine has been reported, e.g, in *Alstonia, Andira, Anomospermum, Aquilegia, Archangelica, Argemone, Berberis, Bocconia, Caltha, Chelidonium, Coelocline, Coptis, Corydalis, Coscinium, Dicentra, Dicranostigma, Enantia, Eschscholzia, Evodia, Fagara, Glaucium, Hunnemannia, Macleaya, Jeffersonia, Leontice, Mahonia, Nandina, Nectandra, Orixa, Papaver, Phellodendron, Platystemon, Podophyllum, Sanguinaria, Thalictrum, Tinospora, Toddalia,*

Vepris, Xanthorrhiza, Xylopia, and *Zanthoxylum*, to mention a few genera. Berberine, still found in certain patent medicines and prescription drugs, has the following activities listed in the FNF (Father Nature's Farmacy) data base: amebicide, analgesic, anticonvulsant, antidiarrheal, antitumor, antiulcer, astringent, bactericide, candidicide, cardiodepressant, carminative, choleretic, collyrium, febrifuge, fungicide, hemostat, hypotensive, immunostimulant, myocardiodepressant, protisticide, RNA-depressant, sedative, stomachic, trypanocide, uterotonic and viricide. If berberine is what we are after, there are weeds, like barberries and prickly poppies, or cultivars like the celandine, California, or plume poppies, we could attack rather than goldenseal. Growing several of these species at my Herbal Village, I am trying to catalyze clinical studies of the barberry, a notorious weed here in the US, as an herbal alternative to the endangered goldenseal. It would be a doubled barrelled approach, decimating a weed while taking the pressure off an endangered species.

Sanguinarine, another rather widely distributed alkaloid, occurs in, e.g., *Argemone, Bocconia, Chelidonium, Corydalis, Dicentra, Dicranostigma, Eschscholzia, Fumaria, Glaucium, Hunnemannia, Hypecoum, Macleaya, Meconopsis, Papaver, Platystemon, Robinia (?), Romneya (?), Sanguinaria, Sapindus (?), Scabiosa (?),* and *Stylophorum*. The bloodroot, *Sanguinaria canadensis*, even made TV last year in commercials for an antiplaque toothpaste. This pleased some ethnobotanists while alarming some conservationists and consumers. Consumers were alarmed that the sanguinarine might poison us, even though Amerindians had used the bloodroot orally as an antiseptic. Conservationists were alarmed that the demand for sanguinarine might endanger the woodland bloodroot. Sanguinarine is not a non-toxic alkaloid. Still it was being put in toothpaste to control plaque. The TV ads showed handsome toothsome ladies with bright smiles and holding the Sanguinaria root. Those smiles have disappeared from my TV screen. I'm told the FDA has challenged the manufacturers to prove that sanguinarine is both safe and efficacious for the prevention of plaque. Should there be a demand for sanguinarine, it might better be supplied by some of our cultivars than by the diminutive bloodroot. In some tropical "Extractive Reserves" there are species of *Bocconia* which behave like weed trees. These might prove more reliable renewable sources of sanguinarine, taking the pressure off our delightful bloodroot.

German immunological research may increase pressure on our *Echinacea's*, some of which are common, others of which are under review for listing, e.g., *Echinacea laevigata* or *Echinacea tennesseensis* (DOI, 1985). The German research puts the coneflower in the lead among American immunomodulatory herbs, ranking up there with Chinese *Astragalus membranaceus*, on sale in New York as "huang qui" as an immune booster. Incidentally, there were nearly two pages of Astragali proposed for listing (DOI, 1985). Kindscher (1989) reports recent pharmacological studies showing that a daily dose of 10 mg/kg of coneflower polysaccharide is effective as an immunostimulant. But higher dosages result in "markedly decreased pharmacological activity". As early as 1902, long before the interest in immunomodulators, Kansas yielded up 200,000 pounds of the "Kansas Snakeroot" worth over $100,000. Concern over their status led Missouri in 1987 to outlaw the harvest of *E. pallida, E. purpurea* and *E. paradoxa* on state parkland, highways, state forest lands, and wildlife areas. The "Missouri Snakeroot", *Parthenium integrifolium,* was used as a weedy adulterant of the Kansas snakeroot, even in the German studies showing the immunostimulant activity (Foster, 1989). But this turns out to be more good news for

Parthenium than bad news for Echinacea. Both have immunostimulant activity. In my data base (Duke 1992a,b), now available online at: http://www.ars-grin.gov/~ngrlsb/ flowers of *Echinacea* are the best apparent source of cichoric acid, an integrase inhibitor that may be exploited for the treatment of AIDS. That news may put increasing pressure on *Echinacea*.

Some people are concerned that there might be endangerment of the trailing arbutus *(Epigaea repens)*, which often shares its habitat with the pink ladyslipper, pipsissewa and wintergreen. All these ericads contain arbutin (Foster and Duke, 1990), which the Merck Index describes as a diuretic urinary antiseptic. This might explain their long folk use for urogenital ailments, especially cystitis. The Merck Index (8th ed) adds: "Gallotannin (also in ericads) prevents enzymes such as B-glucosidase from splitting arbutin which explains why crude plant extracts are more effective medicinally than pure arbutin. In my neighborhood (Howard Co, Md), the trailing arbutus is common while *Chimaphila umbellate* and *Gaultheria procumbens* are uncommon. None of these transplant well, and their medicinal use may be on the decline. I suspect that wild flower diggers may "endanger" these more than herbalists. At one time, the methyl-salicylate industry put pressure on wintergreen, but the cherry birch proved a much better source of methyl-salicylate, now largely if not wholly synthetic. One Canadian boy died last year after ingesting wintergreen oil (NMH Herb Market Review, p. 13. Spring 1990). I suspect a teaspoon of almost any pure essential oil could be lethal.

Another aromatic medicinal is the American pennyroyal, *Hedeoma pulegioides*. By no means endangered itself, it does have quite a medicinal folklore, and more importantly, its active ingredient, pulegone, is being studied as an insect repellent. If pulegone repels ants, birds, caterpillars, fleas, and ticks as some claim, you can anticipate increased interest in species that contain it. Assuming that *Hedeoma todsenii,* known only from two populations in New Mexico, and *Dicerandra immaculate,* endangered central Florida scrub species, both contain pulegone, we have two Center for Plant Conservation (CPC) Priority "All endangered species" in two genera of the Lamiaceae. Four *Dicerandra's* and 9 *Hedeoma's* are proposed for listing (DOI, 1985). Not to worry? Yes! Worry about these species! They might have isomers or compounds somewhat different to pulegone with greater biological activities.

Working with *Dicerandra frutescens,* Thomas Eisner (Eisner et al, 1990) found just such a compound, (+)-trans-pulegol, "a new natural product ... which stands out as the major defensive compound of this mint" , along with 1,8-cineole, isomenthol, isomenthone, 3,8-menthadiene, 2,4(8)menthadiene, menth-3-en-8-ol, neomenthol, alpha pinene, beta-pinene, pulegone and sabinene. Endangered species can contain new natural products, useful to man, or they many contain genes with which to improve the agronomic potential of less endangered species! But don't worry about the pulegone itself! Father Nature has been kind and spread the pulegone around. Pulegone is reported, e.g., in *Barosma, Capsicum, Dicerandra, Hedeoma, Lycopus, Mentha, Monarda, Nepeta, Pycnanthemum, Satureja, Schizonepeta, and Teucrium*. I have a *Pycnanthemum* which smells strongly of pulegone, which grows to nearly 2 m tall, spreads rapidly and produces hundreds of seed. I'll bet it will produce 100 times as much pulegone per hectare as *Hedeoma pulegioides* produces. Although pulegone has anticholinesterase activity that might prove useful in

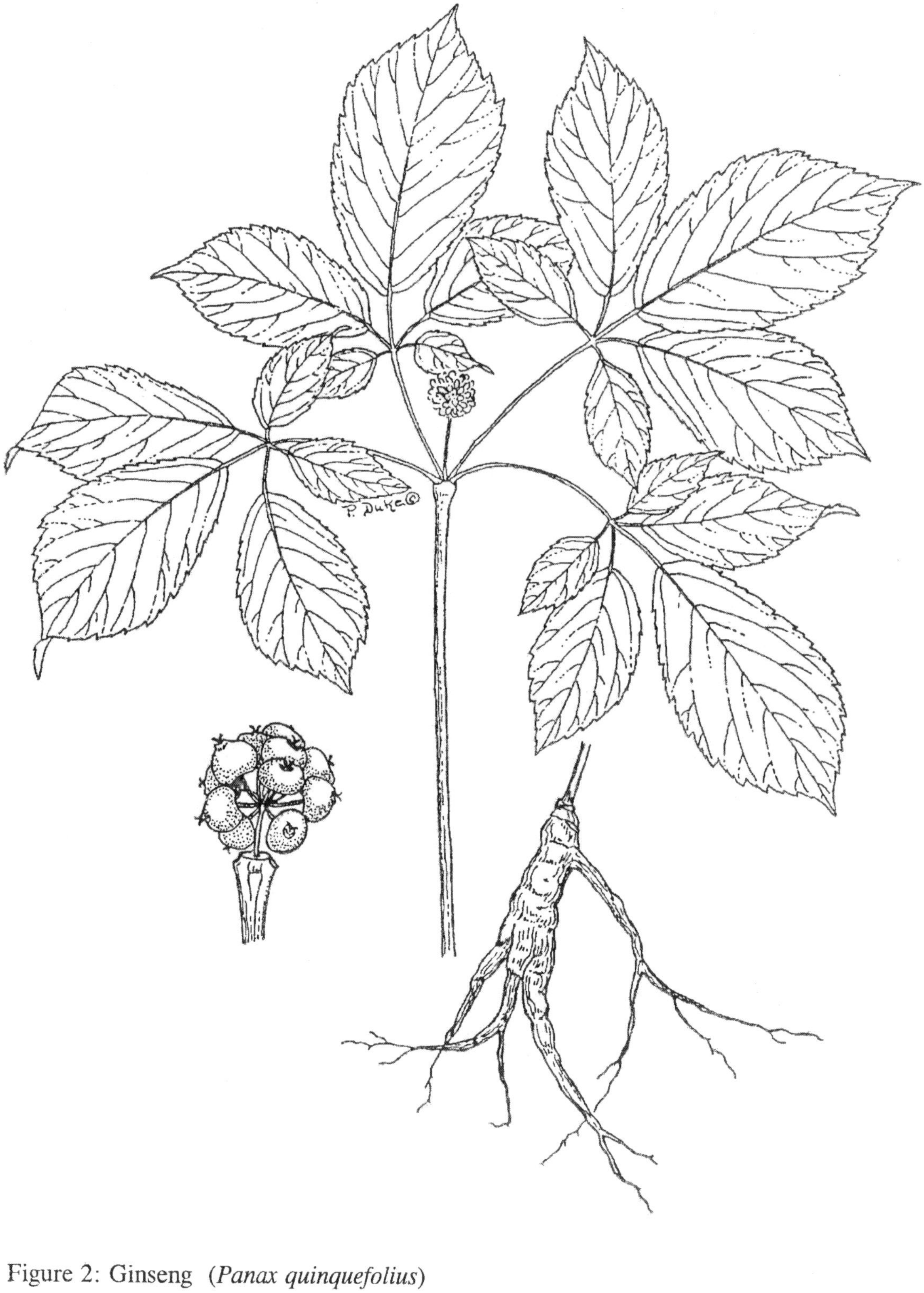

Figure 2: Ginseng (*Panax quinquefolius*)

Alzheimer's disease, like the anticholinesterase activity of Cognex (Tacrine), pulegone has also been shown to have hepatocarcinogenic and hepatotoxic activities. It is absorbed through the skin, so even its insect-repelling qualities may have negative health consequences.

Father Nature was not so generous with taxol. It occurs, e.g., in the bark of the western yew, *Taxus brevifolia*, a slow growing forest tree that may be 24 m tall. Even there, taxol occurs in very small quantities (100 ppm). Trees can provide 5-20 pounds of bark. Alice Christen of the USDA once told me that it would take 2,000-4,000 trees to provide one kilogram of taxol (enough for clinical trials on 500-1000 people). The western yew is a giant, compared to our eastern yew, *Taxus canadensis*. One eastern yew I collected in the North Woods of Maine had ~500 ppm in the renewable needles. The most endangered perhaps is *Taxus floridana*, almost extinct in the wild in Florida. Taxol also occurs at levels of 20-700 ppm in the needles and 10-90 ppm in stems of *Taxus baccata, T. brevifolia, T. canadensis, T. cuspidata, and T. media*. (Gordon Cragg, NCI, pers. comm., Apr 10, 1990). Although taxol has been produced in tissue culture, and a fungus can produce it, and although it has been synthesized, I predict that in the year 2000, when sales will approximate a billion US dollars a year, that taxol will still be largely produced by extraction from yews, cultivated or wild. Taxol shows great promise in ovarian cancer. Oncologists working with taxol regard it as one of the best new anticancer agents around. It is the only plant product known to promote the assembly of microtubules and inhibit the tubulin disassembly process.

Growing in the forest with my volunteer *Taxus* seedlings is an even more "primitive" plant, the shining clubmoss, *Lycopodium lucidulum*. This may well be our occidental analog of oriental *Huperzia serrata*, source of the anticholinesterase alkaloids, huperzine A and B. Based on the morphological similarities of the two species, I predicted we would find anticholinesterase activity, if not huperzine, in our American species. Dr. Alan Kozikowski, then Professor of Chemistry at the U. Pittsburg, and now with the Mayo Clinic in Florida, analyzed my material of *L. lucidulum*, and concluded that there was no huperzine therein, although there was a chromatographic peak at the same place as the huperzine peak in *H. serrata*. Kozikowski also advised me that selagine from *Lycopodium selago* is identical with huperzine. Thus, we do have huperzine in America, in *L. selago*, common in North America, but perhaps not so easily transplantable. I now have three species of *Lycopodium* transplanted into my forest, and know where to find material of 5-6 other species nearby, if there are chemists wishing to compare their anticholinesterase activity with that of sav'ry, sage, rosemary and thyme, also apparently promising in Alzheimer's. Huperzine is supposed, by optimists I think, to have three times the anticholinesterase activity of phytostigmine (the important alkaloid physostigmine is derived from Africa's *Physostigma*, of which we have none in the US). Even the condom industry puts a little pressure on other species of *Lycopodium*. Balick & Beitel (1989) note that "one major brand of non-lubricated condoms was coated with spores of the staghorn clubmoss, *Lycopodium clavatum*, spores 'of known hazardous nature'. Used previously in the manufacture of diverse products including hair powder, suppositories, and surgical gloves, these spores have caused allergic reactions ranging from hay fever to more serious giant cell granulomas. This foreign body response can stimulate neoplastic disease, tuberculosis, or syphilis". That kind of press may reduce the pressure, for *Lycopodium* spores at least. I am actively seeking spores of *Lycopodium selago*, trying to get the species into tissue culture.

Substitution among medicinal plants: the case of ginseng

Substitution of one medicinal plant with another, or competition among different plants for the same medicinal use, often occurs. An interesting example is ginseng. Conservationists tell me that ginseng, our number 1 crude medicinal export at ca $50 million a year, is being eradicated by collection from the wild. West Virginians and western Marylanders tell me that's not the case, that there is plenty of ginseng, that the armchair botanists don't get far enough off the roads. Certainly the Chinese, importers of most of our ginseng exports, have all but wiped out their own ginseng in the wild. They are vigorously cultivating both *Panax ginseng* and *Panax quinquefolius,* to such a degree that someday they may endanger our ginseng trade, thereby ironically taking some of the pressure off our ginseng. But not completely. Chinese buyers still pay much less for cultivated ginseng, than for the wild, which they believe has more activity. Cultivated ginseng is usually priced "75 to 80 percent below" the wild. Thus, demand for wild American ginseng will probably continue to put stress on natural populations in North America (Singer, 1990). The Chinese have sometimes sold *Eleutherococcus senticosus* as a poor man's substitute for ginseng and Russian exporters are promoting the species as an adaptogen and immunostimulant. This so-called Siberian ginseng is a spiny, rhizomatous weedy understory shrub that grows in the forest of Siberia and northern China. A few enthusiasts in America have introduced the species. Without its native enemies, it may someday take off to compete with the honeysuckle and multiflora rose, invading some of the little remaining ginseng habitat. While this Siberian ginseng may take a little pressure off the American ginseng today, it may become its deadly enemy in the 21st century.

It seems appropriate to close this discussion with ginseng, America's most famous "medicinal herbal export". Many males consume ginseng in the questionable belief that it is an aphrodisiac. They even cite the population statistics of China to support their contention. Some might even suggest: "The more ginseng, the more babies". That is lamentable. I feel that population pressure is what endangers species the most. As we try to feed more and more people, forests are felled and converted to agroecosystems, further endangering the forest species thru habitat reduction. The better the medicinal plant, the more it threatens its own existence, first by the people who use it and live longer, and second by the collectors who provide the raw materials. I wish to paraphrase what centenarian Dr. R. R. Stewart said at the Plant Life Symposium in his honor at Karachi: "If you want to conserve plants, you must practice family planning. If you insist on having children, you must teach them. It's much more difficult to teach children than to have them". I'm afraid the bottom line reads, the more people we have, the fewer medicinal plants we'll have to maintain their health. Maybe Gaia will get even with us.

In my backyard in Maryland's eastern deciduous forest, there are four species, three native and frost tolerant, one exotic and frost-sensitive species, that could be or are used as starter materials for four billion dollar drugs. They are *Dioscorea villosa* for steroids, long a billion dollar a year industry, *Podophyllum peltatum,* possible starter for etoposide, 1996 sales ca 400 million, *Taxus* species, all of which contain taxol in their needles, taxol's sales in 1996 ca 600 million, and *Catharanthus roseus*, for nearly 4 decades source of vincristine and vinblastine, average sales often exceeding 100 million per year. We find starter materials for four different billion dollar drugs in my small piece of the relatively depauperate eastern deciduous forest. How many billion dollar drugs are still waiting for us in the e.g. "ACEER forest" (Amazonian Center for Environmental Education and Research, off the Napo Ricer in Amazonian Peru, with 300 woody species per hectare). How many of these do we lose before they are even named if we allow such forests to disappear? How many have potential drugs for today's killer diseases, developing resistance to our last-defense antibiotics like vancomycin? How many have potential for other diseases, even some diseases unknown today, of the future?

"Axeman leave that tree alone; the life you spare may be your own!"

References

Balick, M. J. and Beitel, J. M. 1989. Lycopodium Spores Used in Condom Manufacture: Associated Health Hazards. Econ. Bot. 43(3): 373-7.

DOI. 1985. Endangered and Threatened Wildlife and Plants; Review of Plant Taxa for Listing as Endangered or Threatened Species; Notice of Review. Federal Register Part IV. Dept. of Interior. Fish and Wildlife Service. Sept. 27, 1985. USGPO, Washington.

Duke, J.A. 1988. Should the Forest Disappear. HerbalGram 17:23, Summer.

Duke, J.A. 1989. Ginseng, a Concise Handbook. 273 pp. Reference Publications, Box 344, Algonac, MI 48001.

Duke, J.A. 1992. CRC Handbook of Edible Weeds, CRC Press, Inc., 2000 Corporate Blvd., N.W., Boca Raton, FL 33431. 256 pp.

Duke, J.A. 1992a. CRC Handbook of Phytochemical Constituents in GRAS Herbs and other Economic Plants. CRC Press, Boca Raton, FL 33431. 654 pp. (Available on diskette with manual)

Duke, J.A. 1992b. CRC Handbook of Biologically Active Phytochemicals and Their Activities. CRC Press, Boca Raton, FL 33431. 183 pp. (Available on diskette with manual.)

Duke, J.A. 1993. You, Yew, and Biofuel. Maine Naturalist 1(2):21-30.

Duke, J.A. 1994. Herbal Stamps That Should Have Been. The Herb Companion. April/May:72-76.

Duke, J. A. 1997. The Green Pharmacy. Rodale Press, Emaus PA 18098-0099. 507 pp.

Eberhard, W. 1986. Dictionary of Chinese Symbols (Routledge, New York. 332 pp. English translation 1986)

Eisner, T., McCormick, K.D., Sakaino, M., Eisner, M., Smedley, S.R., Aneshansley, D.J., Deyrup, M., Myers, R.L. & Meinwald, J. Chemical defense of a rare mint plant. *Chemoecology* 1:(1) 30-37.

Eisner, T. et al. 1990 in ed. Chemical Defense of a Rare Mint Plant. Submitted for publication in the first issue of Chemoecology.

Foster, S. 1989. Phytogeographic and Botanical Considerations of Medicinal Plants in Eastern Asia and Eastern North America. pp. 115-144 in Craker, L. E. and Simon, J. E., eds. Herbs, Spices, and Medicinal Plants: Recent Advances in Botany, Horticulture and Pharmacology. Vol. 4. Oryx Press, Phoenix. 267 pp.

Foster, S. and Duke, J. A. 1990. A Field Guide to Medicinal Plants: Eastern and Central North America. Houghton Miflin Co. , Boston MASS. (Peterson Field Guide Series #40)

Kindscher, K. 1989. Ethnobotany of Purple Coneflower *(Echinacea angustifolia,* Asteraceae) and other Echinacea species. Econ. Bot. 43(4): 498-507.

Marshall, N. T. 1989. Progress in the Plant Kingdom. Traffic USA 9(4): 7-9.

McCaleb, R. 1990. Botanical Resources Threatened. Herb Market Review. Special Inclosure in Natural Foods Merchandiser. Spring 1990. p 1, 20, 22.

Moerman, D. E. 1986. Medicinal Plants of Native America. U. Mich. Mus. Anthop. Tech. Rept. # 19. 2 vols. Ann Arbor.

Principe, P. P. 1989. The Economic Significance of Plants and Their Constituents as Drugs: pp. 1-17 in Wagner, H., Hikino, H., and Farnsworth, N. R., eds. Economic and Medicinal Plants Research, vol. 3. Academic Press, Orlando FL

Singer, S. R. 1990. Current Status of the U. S. Ginseng Export Program. Endang. Sp. Tech. Bull. 15(l): 9.

Spiller, G. A. Ed. 1996. CRC Handbook of Lipids in Human Nutrition. CRC Press. Boca Raton, FL. 233 pp.